BURT FRANKLIN: RESEARCH & SOURCE WORKS SERIES 628
Science Classics 4

CONTRIBUTIONS

TO THE

ANNALS OF MEDICAL PROGRESS

AND

MEDICAL EDUCATION

CONTRIBUTIONS

TO THE

ANNALS OF MEDICAL PROGRESS

AND

MEDICAL EDUCATION

IN

THE UNITED STATES

BEFORE AND DURING

THE WAR OF INDEPENDENCE

BY

JOSEPH M. TONER, M. D.

BURT FRANKLIN
NEW YORK

Published by LENOX HILL Pub. & Dist. Co. (Burt Franklin)
235 East 44th St., New York, N.Y. 10017
Originally Published: 1874
Reprinted: 1970
Printed in the U.S.A.

S.B.N.: 8337-35470
Library of Congress Card Catalog No.: 73-143662
Burt Franklin: Research and Source Works Series 628
Science Classics 4

Reprinted from the original edition in the University of Pennsylvania Library.

CONTENTS.

	Page.
Letter of the Commissioner of Education to the Secretary of the Interior	5
Introductory	7
Lack of early legislation	7
Reasons of inaction	7
Medical pioneers in Virginia	8
Virginia surgeons in the revolutionary war	10
Medical pioneers in Massachusetts—seventeenth century	12
Medical pioneers in Massachusetts—eighteenth century	22
Massachusetts surgeons in the revolutionary war	35
Miscellanea respecting early medical practice	35
Early medical practice in New York	37
New York physicians of the eighteenth century	42
New York army-surgeons in the Revolution	46
After the Revolution	48
Honors to medical men	49
Small number of trained practitioners	49
Beginnings of legislative protection	49
Rise of hospitals	54
Autopsy	57
Midwifery	58
The physician and the apothecary	58
Fees	58
Medical titles	59
Medicine in the South	61
Carolina surgeons in the Revolution	62
North Carolina	63
Early medical training in New England	64
Connecticut physicians	65
Connecticut surgeons in the Revolution	69
Early physicians in Rhode Island	70
Medical science elsewhere	73
Early physicians in New Jersey	73
Formation of medical societies	77
Early physicians in Pennsylvania	78
Pennsylvania surgeons in the Revolution	83
Pennsylvania Hospital	85
Pest-houses	85
Clinical instruction	85
Medical library of the Pennsylvania Hospital	86
Early physicians in Maryland	86
Maryland surgeons in the Revolution	90
Early physicians of Delaware	91
Georgia surgeons in the Revolution	93
Surgeons not located	93
Surgeons at Bunker Hill	93
Endemics and epidemics	93
Reasons for studying abroad	95

CONTENTS.

	Page.
Founding of medical schools at home	96
Medical College of Philadelphia	96
Early physicians in New Hampshire	100
Medical College of New York	101
Rules of admission and examination	102
Date of first degrees	102
Annual sessions	102
Progress of medical education	102
Interruption from war	109
Alphabetical index to names of physicians mentioned in the text	110

LETTER.

DEPARTMENT OF THE INTERIOR,
BUREAU OF EDUCATION,
Washington, D. C., October 27, 1874.

SIR: I have the honor to recommend the publication of the accompanying manuscript, prepared by J. M. Toner, M. D., founder of the Toner lectures in Washington, a writer on several important medical topics, and president of the American Medical Association.

This compilation of biographical and historical notes concerning the physicians of the colonial times and the early days of American independence was undertaken by Dr. Toner at the request of the Convention of School-Superintendents which met in Washington in 1872, (to consult with regard to the exhibition of the United States system of education at Vienna,) with a view to its forming a part of that complete representation of the rise and progress as well as present condition of the system of education in the United States, professional and preparatory, which was thought desirable for the Vienna Exhibition.

The difficulties attending a compilation from such scattered and varied sources prevented its completion in season for Vienna. Prepared during the intervals of active professional work, it makes no claim to a methodical or exhaustive treatment of the subject; it however furnishes a mass of biographical and historical information now for the first time collected, which must make it a valuable contribution towards a history of the rise and progress of medical culture in this country, and most useful to other inquirers in the same field. Its brief biographies of the early medical practitioners show how often the learned professions were united in the same learned man, who was at once physician, pastor, and teacher, and how medical science was at first traditional, the old practitioner instructing his one or two student-assistants in his own theories and methods and they in turn handing them down, with the added results of their own experience, to their successors.

The importance of correct methods of training for this profession, to whose care more or less directly are committed the lives and health of all our people, cannot be overestimated. This compilation furnishes the first steps for all who would pursue the instructive lessons of experience to their conclusion. It is also specially timely as an aid in presenting at the Centennial Exhibition the growth of this profession during the colonial period of our country's history. It is to be hoped that some equally intelligent and enthusiastic investigator will do for the past century what Dr. Toner has attempted for the period comprised in his own researches.

Very respectfully, your obedient servant,

JOHN EATON,
Commissioner.

Hon. C. DELANO,
Secretary of the Interior.

Approved and publication ordered.

C. DELANO,
Secretary of the Interior.

CONTRIBUTIONS TO THE ANNALS OF MEDICAL PROGRESS AND EDUCATION.

In response to the request of eminent educators, the following records and notes, which I have made, from time to time, on the rise and progress of medical culture during the earliest years of the settlement of this country, are furnished, rather as memoranda for the use of those interested in similar studies, than as an attempt to push investigations to their conclusions or to follow exactness of method.

As the medical profession must always occupy an important, if not a conspicuous, position in the scientific and educational history of a nation, the present is deemed an opportune occasion to group together in a brief review some of the more notable names of medical men and important events in the history and progress of medicine in the United States, from the period of the first settlements to the close of the colonial governments, and in some instances down to the commencement of the present century.

LACK OF EARLY LEGISLATION.

For the first century, after successful settlements had been made on this continent, medicine, as a distinct branch of education, received but little consideration from legislators, and, as a profession and an art, was left wholly without protection, encouragement, or recognition.

The school-house everywhere accompanied the pioneer, and academic institutions promptly sprang up in the interest of the various denominations, and achieved reputation in not less than eight distinct settlements before the Revolution.

But up to this period only two attempts to establish medical colleges had been made, and from these less than fifty young men had been graduated as bachelors and doctors of medicine. Many of the causes influencing this backwardness in home-professional education are apparent in the dependent attitude of the colonies and the state of the profession in both hemispheres.

REASONS OF INACTION.

But few physicians were required by the healthy and laborious people, of steady habits, who first came to our shores. The sparseness of the population, which was gradually subduing the forest and planting settlements on the bays setting up from the Atlantic and along the rivers emptying into them, gave but little encouragement to the professional man.

So intently occupied were the first immigrants with the struggle to obtain the necessaries of life, surrounded as they were by unfriendly tribes of natives and in a rigorous climate, that they had no time to think of medical education or medical matters, however important these things might be to the preservation of their health and the securing of final success in their endeavors.

Education, particularly professional, requires means and leisure for its encouragement and a reasonable prospect of remunerative employment. It is true, the immediate wants of the colonists, arising from sickness or accidents, were in a measure provided for by physicians who accompanied the early pioneers of civilization to these shores.

MEDICAL PIONEERS IN VIRGINIA.

Among the early settlers that came to Virginia and founded Jamestown in 1607 was Dr. Thomas Wootton,[1] surgeon-general of the Company. The doctor was among those who suffered severely from lack of food, living for a considerable time on crabs and sturgeon.[2] In 1608 Dr. Walter Russell is mentioned as being with Captain Smith and rendering him professional services during the making of the survey of Chesapeake Bay and the Potomac River. He attended an Indian chief,[3] who had been shot in the knee, a brother of Hassininga, king of one of the four nations of the Mannahocks.

This expedition, consisting of Captain Smith, Dr. Russell, and thirteen of the crew, after surveying the Chesapeake Bay, proceeded up the Potomac River to the Falls, some few miles above where now stands Washington City, the Capital of the United States.

In 1608 Anthony Bagnall[4] was surgeon at the fort and for the settlers at Jamestown and vicinity. Some idea of the special perils attending a professional life in the New World at that day may be inferred from the fact that on one of his visits to a patient he was shot at by the Indians, the arrow passing through his hat.

The residence of these physicians is presumed not to have been permanent, as Captain Smith, the president of the Virginia Company, returned to England in 1609 for surgical treatment, "for there was neither chirurgeon nor chirurgery at the fort."[5]

Dr. Lawrence Bohun studied his profession in the Low Countries, where the leading medical schools of that period were located, and found his way to Virginia as early as 1610, and in 1611 is mentioned as physician-general of the colony. In March of that year, Lord Delaware, who was seriously ill, sailed from Virginia to the West Indies for his health, accompanied by Dr. Bohun. The doctor was killed in a naval engagement with a Spanish man-of-war,[6] and was succeeded in office by Dr. John Pot,[7] who was elected (on the recommendation of Dr. Gulstone) physician-general of the Company, and the same year removed to the colony, of which he was made temporary governor in 1628.[8]

---

[1] Stith's History of Virginia, p. 48.　　[2] Stith's History of Virginia, p. 62.
[3] Stith's History of Virginia, p. 71.　　[4] Stith's History of Virginia, p. 74.
[5] Stith's History of Virginia, p. 106.　　[6] Stith's History of Virginia, p. 188.
[7] Stith's History of Virginia, p. 188.
[8] History of the Virginia Company of London, p. 182.

These were some of the physicians of distinction, and I might add the names of others who practiced in Virginia before the Pilgrims landed at Plymouth.[1]

Dr. Green practiced in Gloucester County, Virginia, and died in 1676, in the same house where General Bacon, of Bacon's rebellion, died. Many of the early physicians who came to Virginia, as well as those who first came to the other colonies, held some official position, either at a fort with the army or in the navy of the country governing the settlements. It is also a noticeable fact that many of the ships, perhaps all, trading with the settlements in the New World in the seventeenth century, carried with them a surgeon. This was rendered necessary on account of the length of the voyage and the time expended in disposing of and collecting new cargoes. These surgeons were permitted while the ships were in port to practice among the people on shore. When the encouragement was sufficient, no doubt some of them remained or, returning, resided permanently.

Dr. William Cabell, a native of Great Britain, was educated to the profession of medicine; came to America between 1720 and 1724. He settled on the James River, at a place known as Liberty Hall, in Nelson County, and was a man of enterprise, wealth, and of great influence in the State. He died April 12, 1774, aged 87.

The earliest law passed having special reference to the medical profession was "An act to compel physicians and surgeons to declare on oath the value of their medicines," enacted October 21, 1639, which was revised and amended at the session of 1645-'46, and again at the session of 1657-'58. (Hening's Stat. Va., vol. i, pp. 316, 450.)

John Mitchell, M. D., F. R. S., removed from England to Virginia about the year 1700 and located at Urbana, a small town on the Rappahannock River. He was eminent as a botanist, as well as a physician; and, besides numerous communications to the Royal Society, he published a work on botany, a history of the contest in America, (printed in 1755,) and a treatise on the yellow fever. The manuscript of the latter having fallen into the hands of Dr. Franklin, he transmitted it to Dr. Rush, at the time that yellow fever was epidemic in Philadelphia; and, from the valuable suggestions contained in it, Dr. Rush was led into a new train

---

[1] Upon examining the colonial laws and enactments, I find the following statutes relating to medicine and hygiene enacted in the colony of Virginia prior to the establishment of the present form of government, the titles only of which have been introduced as affording interest to the reader: An act regulating chirurgeons' accounts, enacted 1662, Hen. Stat. Va., vol. 2, p. 109; An act allowing chirurgeons' accounts to be pleaded after decease of the party, enacted 1662, Hen. Stat. Va., vol. 2, p. 109; An act relating to physicians' and chirurgeons' accounts, enacted 1691, manuscript-ed. Stat. Va., p. 15; An act to oblige ships coming from places infected with plague to perform their quarantine, enacted 1722, Stats. Va., ed. 1769, p. 67; An act for regulating the fees and accounts of the practitioners of physic, enacted 1736, Hen. Stat. Va., vol. 4, p. 509; An act to regulate the inoculation of small-pox within the colony, enacted 1769, Stat. Va., ed. 1785, p. 11; An act amendatory to the foregoing act, enacted 1777, Stat. Va., ed. 1785, p. 164.

of reflections which resulted in his successfully combating the distemper in Philadelphia in 1793. Dr. Mitchell died about 1772.

James Craik, M. D., came to America, probably with Braddock's army, and served as a surgeon throughout the French and Indian war. He was born in Scotland in 1730 and was educated for the medical staff of the British army. He was with General Braddock at the time of his defeat and assisted in dressing his wounds. While in the army, he formed with General (then Colonel) Washington an acquaintance which ripened into a friendship that continued through life.

At the breaking out of the revolutionary war, Dr. Craik tendered his services to the American Army and after the surrender of Yorktown was appointed director-general of the hospital at that place. At the close of the war he was persuaded by Washington to settle at Alexandria, near Mount Vernon. He remained the physician and friend of the general, and was with him at the time of his death. To him Washington refers in his will, calling him "my compatriot in arms; my old and intimate friend." He died in Fairfax County, Virginia, February 6, 1814.

Dr. Walter McClurg was a successful practitioner in Elizabeth City, Va., about the middle of the year 1750.

Hugh Mercer, a native of Scotland, was educated as a physician, and, having emigrated to this country, settled in Virginia. He served in the French and Indian war and, being wounded at Fort Du Quesne, barely escaped capture by the enemy. He entered the American Army at the commencement of the Revolution, and, having distinguished himself in various battles, was made brigadier-general. During the action at Princeton, on the 3d of January, 1777, while endeavoring to rally his retreating troops, his horse was shot from under him and he severely wounded by the British troops, who surrounded and stabbed him with their bayonets. He died January 19, 1777, and was buried at Philadelphia.

Dr. John Spencer was born and educated in Scotland. He was an alumnus of the University of Edinburgh. Arriving in America towards the close of the last century, he settled at Dumfries, Va., where he obtained a large and lucrative practice.

Dr. Andrew Leiper was a resident of Richmond, where he died, October 17, 1798.

VIRGINIA SURGEONS IN THE REVOLUTIONARY WAR.

The following physicians of Virginia served in the Continental Army in their professional capacity, as I find from the historical records of the Revolution:

Cornelius Baldwin, Thomas Chrystie, Mace Clements, Joseph Davis Charles Land, Baziel Middleton, George Monroe, Robert Rose, Joseph, Savage, Alexander Skinner, Nathan Smith, John Tresvant, Claiborne Vaughn, James Wallace, and George Yates.

Surgeon David Gould died July 12, 1781.

William Graham was surgeon's mate of Colonel Alexander Spottswood's regiment.

James McClurg, M. D., a native of Virginia, graduated in medicine from the University of Edinburgh in 1770. He practiced at Richmond, Va., and established his name as a surgeon of high repute in the revolutionary war.

Dr. Alexander Lajournade was commissioned surgeon's mate, March 15, 1778, to Col. Charles Harrison's Virginia and Maryland Artillery.

Dr. Robert Macry was surgeon in the Eleventh Virginia Regiment, November 13, 1776.

Dr. Shuball Pratt was surgeon in the Virginia Line, March 12, 1778.

Dr. John Roberts was appointed surgeon's mate in 1776 and promoted to surgeon the following year.

Dr. Jonathan Calvert was commissioned surgeon's mate November 30, 1776, in Col. Charles Harrison's Virginia and Maryland regiment of artillery.

Dr. James Carter, of Williamsburg, Va., was in 1765 complimented by a vote of thanks and £50, by the president of William and Mary College in Virginia, for his valuable services to the professors and students when they were suffering from the small-pox.

Dr. William Carter, a native of Virginia, pursued his profession at Richmond, Va., where he died, 1798. He was surgeon to the hospital located at Williamsburg, Va., during the revolutionary war.

Dr. Thomas Chrystie served in the capacity of surgeon from April 1, 1778, to the close of the war.

John Clayton, a native of England, was educated to the profession of medicine, came to America early in the eighteenth century, and settled to practice in Gloucester County, Va., where he spent the remainder of his life, dying December 15, 1773. He was eminent in his profession and one of the leading botanists of the time.

Dr. Stephen Cooke was a surgeon in the revolutionary war and was taken prisoner and sent to Bermuda, where he married. He returned to Virginia, and practiced in Loudoun County, Va., until his death, which occurred March, 1816.

James Currie, a native of Scotland, received his diploma at Edinburgh. He emigrated, and practiced with reputation his profession for a long series of years at Richmond, Va., where he died April 23, 1803, aged 63.

Dr. John Baynham was a practitioner of note in Caroline County, Va., during the early and middle part of the eighteenth century.

Dr. William Baynham acquired distinction as a surgeon in Virginia. He resided most of his life in Essex County, dying in the year 1814, aged 65.

Dr. John Minson Galt, of Williamsburg, Va., was a physician of eminence. He was the first physician placed in charge of the lunatic-asylum established by the State in that town. He occupied the position of surgeon in the hospital located there during the revolutionary war. Some of his descendants have distinguished themselves in medicine.

Dr. Cabin Griffin, born in Virginia of Welsh descent, practiced in Yorktown.

His brother, Cyrus Griffin, was the last president of the Continental Congress.

Dr. Joseph Harding practiced with success at Portsmouth, Va., during the latter half of the eighteenth century.

Dr. Walter Jones, a native of Virginia, a physician of brilliant powers and abilities, practiced in Northumberland County, Va. He died in 1815, aged 70.

Dr. Ezekiel Bull, of Virginia, was a surgeon in the Revolution. He died, in 1819, at a very advanced age.

David Griffith was commissioned by the Continental Congress surgeon and chaplain of Colonel William Heth's regiment and was authorized to draw pay in both capacities.

Surgeon William Rumney received from the State of Virginia a grant of six thousand acres of land in recognition of his services, as did also Surgeon Charles Taylor.

To this list of worthies might be added a host of others who served with distinction in Virginia during the colonial and revolutionary wars.

MEDICAL PIONEERS IN MASSACHUSETTS—SEVENTEENTH CENTURY.

Dr. Samuel Fuller, the first physician and surgeon in New England, came to Massachusetts in the Mayflower. He died in 1633, at Plymouth, of a distemper contracted while attending patients suffering from a contagious disease. His wife at a later period was held in esteem as a midwife.[1]

A little later we find the names of other physicians who practiced the healing art throughout the colony. Giles Firmin practiced in Boston in 1634. In 1638 he received a grant of 120 acres of land at Ipswich.

John Fisk[2] settled at Salem in 1637, and was not only a physician but also school-teacher and clergyman.

Dr. William Gager accompanied Governor Winthrop to Boston, where he practiced many years, and his death was the cause of much regret to the good people of Boston.

Dr. Comfort Starr, originally of Cambridge, removed to Duxbury, Plymouth County, in 1638, and then to Boston, where he died in 1660.

Samuel Bellingham and Henry Salstonstall,[3] graduates of Harvard in 1642, studied medicine and received the degree of M. D. in European universities.

Leonard Hoar, M. D., an alumnus of the Harvard class of 1650, received his medical degree in Europe. He also studied theology, and

---

[1] Russell's Recollections of the Pilgrims, p. 246.
[2] Felt's Annals of Salem, p. 427.
[3] Thacher's Medical Biog., pp. 17, 18.

settled as a minister in Sussex, England, but was rejected for nonconformity. He was subsequently for two years president of Harvard College, having been elected in 1672, shortly after his return to America. He died at Quincy, November 28, 1675, aged 45 years.

John Glover, having graduated at Harvard in 1650, went to Europe, where he received his medical degree at Aberdeen, Scotland. On his return he settled as a physician at Roxbury.

Isaac Chancy and John Rogers, qualified as ministers, also received their medical degrees in Europe and on their return to America engaged chiefly in the ministry. The latter was president of Harvard College (at which institution he had graduated in 1649) from 1682 to 1684, when he died, aged 53 years.

Charles Chauncy, who was appointed president of Harvard College in 1654, had a medical education. He retained that position until his death, in 1672. Six of his sons, educated at the college, studied medicine.

Matthew Fuller practiced medicine in Plymouth from 1640 to 1653, when he removed to Barnstable, at which place he died in 1678. He was surgeon-general of the provincial forces in 1673.

Thomas Starrs, of Yarmouth, as early as 1640 was styled chirurgeon·

Samuel Seabury, chirurgeon in Duxbury from an early date, died in 1680.

Thomas Oliver [1] was in practice in Boston about 1640.

In March, 1629, John Pratt was proposed to the court of assistants in London as a surgeon to the Salem Plantations, upon the following conditions: "That £40 should be allowed him: for his chest, £25, and the residue for his own salary for the first year." [2]

At the same meeting the company agreed with Robert Morley, servant of Mr. Andrew Mathews, late barber-surgeon,[3] to serve the company in New England three years, the first year to have twenty nobles, &c. It is much to the credit of those connected with these early settlements in America, that, in most, if not all of them, provisions were made to give succor to the sick.

---

[1] Winthrop's Journal.

[2] Felt's Annals of Salem, vol. 1, p. 62.

[3] The person entitled to the appellation of surgeon in ancient times, as at present, is often also entitled to that of physician, as is the custom with medical officers in military service.

The term "surgery," or "chirurgery," is derived from the Greek $\chi\varepsilon\acute{\iota}\rho$, the hand, and $\check{\varepsilon}\rho\gamma o\nu$, work, and has been applied to that branch of medicine which effects cures through manipulations, the use of instruments, appliances, topical remedies. In the earliest times of which we have an account, the surgeon was an assistant to the physician, the former exercising his art under the direction of the latter. But it early became separated, as, in the oath of Hippocrates, it appears lithotomy was forbidden to the physician. The Arabian physicians thought it beneath their dignity to perform surgical operations. The Romans left this practice to their slaves. Medicine in the infancy of every people or nation is found in the hands of the priests and is largely mixed up with superstitious rites. In Egypt, India, China, Japan, and among savages and even half-civilized tribes in different countries, the healing art is always largely associated

John Clarke, an English physician of eminence, came to Boston in 1638, where he died, in 1664, at the age of 66. An oil-portrait of him is in the possession of the Massachusetts Historical Society.

His eldest son, John Clarke, also a physician, died at Boston, in 1690.

John Wilson, son of Rev. John Wilson, pastor of the first church

---

with the supernatural. The earliest surgeons of which there is any record were the Egyptian priests; and Mr. Kenrick says that "on the walls of the ruined temples of Thebes *basso-relievos* have been found displaying surgical operations and instruments not far different from some in use in modern times." The skill of the early physicians in embalming the bodies of the dead is conceded by all historians to have been great. In Greece, surgery is as old as her mythical period of history. According to Grecian poets, fifty years before the Trojan war, (1242 B. C.,) Melampus, Chiron, and his disciple Esculapius, accompanied an expedition as surgeons. In the Trojan war two sons of Esculapius—Machaon and Podalirius—took care of the wounded Greeks. Venesection and circumcision were among the earliest surgical operations of which we have any account. The Asclepiades are represented as descendants or followers of Esculapius, the son of Apollo, who was deified on account of his great skill in medicine, about fifty years before the Trojan war. Damocedes was eminent as a surgeon, (600 B. C.,) and, being taken prisoner by the Persians, reduced the dislocated ankle of Darius and cured the cancerous breast of his queen, Atosa, after the Egyptian physicians had failed. As might be expected, the want of exact anatomical knowledge retarded progress. The founding of the Alexandria school, under Ptolemy, (300 B. C.,) led to the study of anatomy. Herophilus and Erasistratus were eminent teachers in this university, and are said to have inaugurated the practice of dissecting the human body. It is probable that the use of the tourniquet, the catheter, the crushing of stone, and the mode of extirpating tumors were invented by them or their pupils. Galen practiced both medicine and surgery at Rome in the latter half of the second century. The history of the advance of surgery in the different countries of Europe since the Christian era is much the same.

The term "barber-surgeon" became common at a time when the art of surgery and the art of shaving were performed in England, France, and other countries by the same person. In former times surgery was ranked as the third branch of medicine.

The title "surgeon" or "chirurgeon" first appears to have been recognized by law in England in 1299. The title "barber-surgeon" is much older, probably originating during the early or Middle Ages among some of the communities of the shaven priesthood, which was for many centuries an educated, numerous, and influential order in France and Great Britain. Long anterior to this period, however, it was common for the art of the surgeon and of the physician to be exercised by the priests. This is evident from the fact that in 993 the fourth Lateran council prohibited the regular clergy from performing any operation in surgery "involving the shedding of blood." Operations with the knife after this were assigned chiefly to seculars and clerks, the chief part naturally falling to the tonsorial craft, who were in daily attendance on the priest-physicians; and the barbers, from their vocation, possessing the necessary skill in the use of sharp instruments, were naturally assigned to this duty, under the direction of the priests. Their ambition and their habit of rendering personal services suited them to perform the duties devolving upon a chirurgeon of that period. The priests were not at that time prohibited from practicing medicine. In 1131 the seventh Lateran council forbade the monks and regular canons pursuing the study of civil law and medicine. But the council of Tours, in 1163, finding that the practice of surgery was still to some extent followed by the clergy, they were positively interdicted from all surgical operations. This regulation still further tended to throw business into the hands of the barber-surgeons and apothecaries. In France a company of barber-sur-

built in Boston, was born in 1621, and graduated from Harvard College, in 1642, at the first class-commencement of that institution. He was shortly afterward installed minister of Medfield, and acted for the community in which he lived, as pastor, school-master, and physician, until his death, August 29, 1691.

geons was formed in 1096. They were at the same time keepers of the baths, and for several centuries retained possession of this branch of medicine.

In Great Britain, early in the fourteenth century, the barber-surgeons became influential as a class and their services important to the kings. The first assembly of the craft in England was composed of Roger Strippe, W. Hobbs, T. Goddard, and Richard Kent, since which time they built their hall in Monkwell street. Entries and records relating to the company from 1309 to 1377 are to be seen in their books at the Guildhall Chamber; also the by-laws of the company in 1387 and an act of Parliament of 1420 relating to the company.

In the second expedition against France, in 1417, Thomas Morestide and William Bredewardyn were empowered by a warrant from the king to press as many surgeons and instrument-makers into their service as they could find in the city of London or elsewhere. The barber-surgeons were once an important company in the city of London, and were then the chief if not the only operating surgeons. This company was formed some time previous to its incorporation, through the influence of Thomas Morestide, esq., one of the sheriffs of London, in 1436. He was chirurgeon to three kings of England, Henry IV, Henry V, and Henry VI, and died in 1450.

Jaques Fries and William Hobbs, physicians to Edward IV in 1461, along with the prince and his brother Gloster, under the patronage of St. Cosme and Damianus, became founders of the corporation or brotherhood, under the name of the Masters or Governors of the Mystery or Commonalty of Barbers of London. The charter bears date February 24, 1461, and has the royal seal in green wax. From this period the barber-surgeons are known to have conducted the business with regularity as a body corporate.

There was a distinction observed in the robe or dress of the chirurgeon proper (who had also studied physic) and the barber-chirurgeon. The former was, therefore, allowed to wear the long robe, or gown, and a particular style of cap.

By virtue of the first act of Parliament, persons (not barbers) were admitted to the practice of surgery without possessing the proper qualifications, so that the surgeons and barbers in the third year of Henry VIII, 1512, obtained an act of Parliament to prevent all such persons from practicing surgery within the city of London and seven miles of the same. This latter condition is a privilege enjoyed and enforced by the Royal College of Physicians of London at the present day. Holbein has commemorated in a fine painting the event of Henry VIII delivering the charter to the barber-surgeons, the court of assistance, and the company. This picture, which is 10 by 6 feet, still in good condition, is preserved in the company's hall in Monkwell street. An engraving of it was made by B. Barron, in 1726, the plate of which is preserved by the company, with many other paintings of historical value to the profession. The surgeons who were present at the reception of the charter occupy positions in the picture and are represented as dressed in gowns trimmed with fur. Their names are painted on their persons. Thomas Vicary, (then master,) John Chambre, William Butts, and J. Alsop, who at the time were past-masters, are placed on the right of the king, who is seated in his royal robes and crowned. On his left are Thomas Vicary, J. Aylef, N. Symson, E. Harman, J. Monforde, J. Pen, N. Alcocke, B. Fereis, W. Tylby, and X. Samon.

T. Vicary is reputed to have been the author of the first work on anatomy written in the English language.

In 1515, the sixth year of Henry VIII's reign, the practicing barbers or surgeons, numbering 19, were, "in consideration of their constant attendance upon patients,

Thomas Boylston, father of the distinguished Dr. Zabdiel Boylston, was born at Watertown, January 26, 1637, and subsequently settled, as a physician and chirurgeon, at Brookline, of which town he was unquestionably the first resident physician. He died in 1695.

The first person executed in Massachusetts Bay Colony was Margaret

---

exempted by Parliament from serving in ward- or parish-offices, but likewise from all military service." The surgeons, increasing in number, in time erected themselves into an independent or separate society from the barbers. Representing to Parliament the embarrassments they were laboring under, the subject was taken under consideration, and, for the mutual interests of each, an act was passed under the appellation of the Masters or Governors of the Mystery or Commonalty of Barbers and Surgeons of London. This act strictly enjoined all persons practicing the art of shaving not to intermeddle with that of surgery, except what belongs to the drawing of teeth; so does it likewise all surgeons from following the practice of shaving.

In 1544 Parliament again took the subject into consideration to promote the practice of surgery and medicine, and to encourage all persons skilled in the nature of herbs, roots, and waters to exert themselves in the exercise thereof for the relief and cure of wounded and distressed objects of compassion; and, among other things, provided for each of the arts of shaving and surgery, "that the said mystery, and all the men of the same mystery of the same city, should be one body and one perpetual community, and that their principals of the same commonalty of the most expert men in the mystery of surgery might, with the assent of twelve, or eight persons at the least, of the same community, every year elect and make out of their community two masters or governors, with authority to make statutes and ordinances for the government of the said mystery," &c.

This act at once united, and at the same time separated, the two crafts, one being commonly called The Barbers of London, the other The Surgeons of London. The company of surgeons built a new and elegant hall in the Old Bailey, where they had a large theater and a dissecting-room for teaching anatomy.

The College of Physicians of London was founded in 1518 and fully established by law in 1523; "that the movers and procurers of so good a fellowship for the safety of the lives of men may be preserved, and the causes that moved the King to grant it may be known, they are both signified to us in the King's letters-patent, where it appeareth that this suit was made by John Chambre, Thomas Lindcre, and Fernandes de Victoria, all the King's physicians; and three other physicians, namely, Nicholas Hallewell, John Francis, and Robert Yearly, and chiefly by the intercession of Cardinal Wolsey, lord chancellor."

On the 15th of August, 1630, Charles I confirmed the rights and privileges granted by former patents and acts of Parliament, and gave to this company the right to make by-laws for the government and order of the society, in such manner and under such restrictions as therein mentioned, and "to make annual elections of masters or governors of the said commonalty, whereof two are to be professors in the art and science of surgery; and also to elect ten of the freemen of the society to be examiners of the surgeons of London during their lives."

The Barber-Surgeons' Company of London possess a curious and valuable memorial in the form of a silver cup, partly gilt, the stem and body representing an oak-tree, from which hang acorns fashioned as little bells. The style is in allusion to the celebrated tree that sheltered Charles at Boscobel. The cover of the cup represents the royal crown of England. The cup was made by order of Charles II and by him presented to the company, Charles, (afterward Sir Charles Scarborough,) chief physician to the King, being the master of the company at the time.

The *barbiers-chirurgeons* were separated from the *barbiers-perruquiers* in France, in the time of Louis XIV, and made distinct corporations.

Jones, a physician and doctress. Being charged with witchcraft, it appeared upon examination "that she had such a malignant touch, as many persons were taken with deafness or vomiting, or other violent pains or sickness; her medicines, though harmless in themselves, yet had extraordinarily violent effects; that such as refused her medi-

---

By the year 1745 it was pretty generally recognized that the two arts which the company professed were foreign to and independent of each other; and by an act of Parliament, (No. 18, George III,) to take effect June 24, 1745, entitled "An act for making the surgeons and barbers of London two distinct and separate corporations," they were so separated.

Lord Thurlow, in the House of Peers, July 17, 1797, in his speech opposing the surgeons' incorporation bill, said that, "by a statute still in force, the barbers and surgeons were each to use a pole. The barbers were to have theirs blue and white, striped, with no other appendage; but the surgeons, whose pole was the same in other respects, were to have a gallipot and a red flag in addition, to denote the particular nature of their vocation."

Anterior to the art of printing, the barbers, or rather the barber-surgeons, are represented in different illuminated manuscripts as using a pole colored red. It is probable that the origin of the pole was from the fact that the barbers, in practicing phlebotomy, caused their patients to extend the arm and grasp a small pole or cane to steady the arm and make the blood flow more freely. Convenience suggested a pole for this special purpose; and, to prevent its being stained, it was painted red. Such a pole was hung out at the door, with the white bandages wound around it, as a symbol of their vocation. This practice, no doubt, led to painting the pole in various colors and stripes, as red and white, blue and white, and, perhaps, red, white, and blue.

Prior to the late rebellion, the colors used on barbers' poles in the United States were red and white only. It is a noticeable fact, however, that the patriotism of the barbers of the country during the war with the South has induced them to adopt almost universally the national colors for their poles, so that now they are mostly striped with red, white, and blue.

In Constantinople the barbers still act as surgeons and dentists, and weave the teeth they have drawn, along with beads, into fanciful designs, and exhibit them at the doors and windows. Some barbers of London, even at the present time, exhibit, in their windows, the teeth they have drawn, as a sign that pulling teeth is a part of their business. During the late war, a barber by the name of Striker had a shop on Seventh street, in Washington City, opposite the Patent-Office, and used to keep hanging at his door and windows, and in several places in his shop, long strings of human teeth that he had drawn, to remind persons that, in addition to shaving and cutting hair, he professed the art of drawing teeth.

There are in the United States but four vocations with which I am acquainted that adopt symbols instead of lettered signs or the exhibition of some implement of their craft or manufacture as a mode of announcing business. These are the barber, the pawnbroker, the tea- and spice-dealer, and the tobacconist. The latter has adopted the figure of an Indian in costume, and is the only one of the four originating in America. The symbol of three balls, which constitutes the pawnbrokers' sign, is taken from the coat of arms of the Medici family, who for centuries were leading physicians in Italy, and subsequently became wealthy bankers, but retained on their coat of arms the sign of three pills, in proud recollection of their ancient vocation. The tea- and spice-dealers have adopted the figure of a Chinese in native costume, indicative of the country from which the goods they offer for sale are brought.

For the information in this note I am indebted to Entick's and also to Allen's History of London, Rowland on the Human Hair, Larwood's History of Sign-boards, and to numerous encyclopedias and other works.

cines she would tell that they would never be healed, and accordingly their diseases and hurts continued with relapses against the ordinary course, and beyond the apprehension of all physicians and surgeons."

Another doctress, a Mrs. Hutchinson, who resided in Boston about the year 1637, had the reputation of being a very skillful midwife. She was banished from the colony, however, for agitating measures against the state.

John Alcock graduated from Harvard in 1646, pursued the study of medicine and practiced in Roxbury, his native town, until his death in 1667, in the forty-second year of his age.

The second physician of Weymouth was Dr. Beal, who began practice there about 1633. Tradition says that his practice and reputation were good.

Samuel Alcock, brother of Dr. John Alcock, was born at Roxbury, and settled at Boston as a chirurgeon. He died March 16, 1677, at the age of 39 years.

Benjamin Tompson, son of Rev. William Tompson, resided at Roxbury, where he enjoyed considerable local celebrity as a physician, schoolmaster, and poet. He was born at Braintree, July 6, 1642, graduated from Harvard in 1662, and died April 13, 1714.

A noted midwife of Boston was Ruth Barnaby, who practiced her calling in that town for more than forty years. She was born at Marblehead, in August, 1664, and died February 12, 1765, aged 101 years. During the revisitation of the small-pox in 1764, although over 100 years old, she insisted on being inoculated, and thus escaped the loathsome disease, notwithstanding several members of her family contracted it.

Robert Child, a native of England, but educated at Padua for the medical profession, immigrated to Massachusetts as early as 1644 and located at Hingham. In 1646 he and others were fined for protesting against the union of the church and state. Dr. Child prepared to sail for Europe, in order to lay his case before Parliament; but the court, anticipating his design, caused him to be apprehended, and, adjudging him guilty of contempt, quadrupled his former fine and ordered his imprisonment until payment was made. His original intention in coming to this country was to explore the mineral resources of the New World. He was a very learned man, for the times, and his bitterest opponent, Governor John Winthrop, spoke of him as " a man of quality, a gentleman, and a scholar."

Among the immigrants to New England in 1650 was Dr. William Avery, a native of England and a subsequent benefactor of Harvard College. He settled at Dedham, but afterward removed to Boston, where he died, March 18, 1686, aged 65 years.

Edward Winslow, at one time governor of Massachusetts, was born in Worcestershire, England, and died of fever, near the isle of Jamaica.

May 8, 1655. It appears that he possessed a knowledge of medicine, "for, having visited Massasoit and finding him very sick, he prescribed for him, curing his affliction, which so pleased the king that he disclosed a plot of the Indians for the destruction of the colony." It is also incidentally mentioned of him that he was at Leyden previous to his immigration to this country.

Daniel Allen, son of Rev. John Allen, the first minister of Dedham, was born in 1656 and graduated from Harvard in 1675. He received a medical education and resided in Boston, where he probably practiced his profession. He was librarian of the college-library at the time of his death, which occurred in 1692.

Jonathan Avery, son of Dr. William Avery, was born in Boston; and in his will, made in May, 1691, he describes himself as "a resident of Dedham, a practitioner of physic, aged 35 years." A tradition existed among the doctor's descendants that he was a believer in alchemy and spent much of his time in chemical studies.

In 1662 Dr. John Touton, a native of Rochelle, in France, applied to the general court of Massachusetts for the privilege of settling in the colony for himself and fellow-Protestants.

Dr. Oliver Noyes, a representative of Boston, died in 1721, aged 48 years. He graduated from Harvard in 1695 and was highly esteemed.

Benjamin Bullivant, a gentleman of noble family, practiced medicine in Boston in 1686, and became distinguished for skill in his profession, and as a pharmacist had no equal in Boston. He was an excellent scholar, was appointed attorney-general, and discharged the trust with credit. He was one of the wardens of the first Episcopal church built in Boston.

Benjamin Ware, a physician of Wrentham, was born in that town July 8, 1688, and died January 18, 1744, much respected as a physician and citizen.

Dr. Nathaniel White was born in Weymouth in 1690 and died in 1758, having held a good reputation and practice and during life discharged several public trusts to the satisfaction of the people.

Dr. Francis Lee Baron practiced medicine in Plymouth from 1693 to 1704, the date of his death.

Nathaniel Phillips resided in Boston at an early date, and kept an apothecary-shop in Orange (now Washington) street, at the corner of Bennet.

Thomas Thacher, (usually spelled Thatcher,) who came to New England in 1635, was educated in medicine as well as theology, and his duties as a physician occupied much of his time. He was made minister of Weymouth in 1644, but accepted a pastorate in Boston at a later period. His professional career is distinguished by the publication, in 1677, of the first contribution to medical literature in America, under the title of a "Brief Rule to Guide the Common People of New England how to

Order themselves and theirs in the Small Pocks, or Measels."[1] Dr. T.

[1] The article is printed in double column, on one side, as a poster, 15½ by 10¼ inches, and reads as follows:

BRIEF RULE

To guide the Common People of

NEW-ENGLAND

How to order themselves and theirs in the

Small Pocks, or Measels.

The *small Pox* (whose nature and cure the *Measels* follow) is a disease in the blood, endeavouring to recover a new form and state.

2. This nature attempts—1. By Separation of the impure from the pure, thrusting it out from the Veins to the Flesh.—2. By driving out the impure from the Flesh to the Skin.

3. The first Separation is done in the first four dayes by a Feaverish boyling (Ebullition) of the Blood, laying down the impurities in the Fleshy parts which kindly effected the Feaverish tumult is calmed.

4. The second Separation from the Flesh to the Skin, or *Superficies* is done through the rest of the time of the disease.

5. There are several Errors in ordering these sick ones in both these Operations of Nature which prove very dangerous and commonly deadly either by overmuch hastening Nature beyond its own pace, or in hindering of it from its own vigorous operation.

6. The Separation by Ebullition in the Feaverish heat is over heightned by too much Clothes, too hot a room, hot *Cordials*, as *Diascordium, Gascons powder* and such like, for hence come *Phrenzies*, dangerous excessive sweats, or the flowing of the Pocks into one overspreading sore, vularly called the Flox.

7. The same seperation is overmuch hindred by preposterous cooling that Feaverish boyling heat, by *blood letting, Glysters, Vomits, purges,* or *cooling medicines.* For though these many times hasten the coming forth of the *Pox*, yet they take away that supply which should keep them out till they are ripe, wherefore they sink in again to the deadly danger of the sick.

8. If a *Phrensie* happen, or through a *Plethorie* (that is fulness of blood) the Circulation of the blood he hiudred, and thereupon the whole mass of blood choaked up, then either let blood, Or see that their diet, or medicines be not altogether cooling, but let them in no wise be heating, therefore let him lye no otherwise covered in his bed than he was wont in health: His Chamber not made hot with fire if the weather be temperate, let him drink small Beer only warm'd with a Tost, let him sup up thin *water-gruel,* or *water-pottage* made only of Indian Flour and water, instead of *Oatmeal:* Let him eat *boild Apples:* But I would not advise at this time any medicine besides. By this means that excessive *Ebullition* (or boyling of his blood) will by degrees abate, and the Symptoms cease; If not, but the blood be so inraged that it will admit no delay, then either let blood (if Age will bear it) or else give some notably cooling medicine, or refresh him with more free Air.

9. But if the boiling of the blood be weak and dull that there is cause to fear it is not able to work a Separation, as it's wont to be in such as have been let blood, or are fat, or Flegmatick, or brought low by some other sickness or labour of the (*Gonorrhea*) running of the Reins, or some other Evacuation: In such Cases, *Cordials* must drive them out, or they must dy.

10. In time of driving out the *Pocks* from the Flesh, here care must be had that the *Pustules* keep out in a right measure till they have attain'd their end without going in again, for that is deadly.

11. In this time take heed when the *Pustules* appear whilst not yet ripe, least by too much heat there arise a new *Ebullition* (or Feaverish boyling) for this troubles the driving out, or brings back the separated parts into the blood, or the Fleshy parts over-heated are disabled from a right suppuration, or lastly the temper of the blood and tone of the Flesh is so perverted that it cannot overcome and digest the matter driven out.

12. Yet on the other hand the breaking out must not be hindred, by exposing the sick unto the cold. The degree of heat must be such as is natural agrees with the temper of the fleshy parts: That which exceeds or falls short is dangerous: Therefore the season of the year, Age of the sick, and their manner of life here require a discreet and different Consideration, requiring the Counsel of an expert Physitian.

13. But if by any error a new *Ebullition* ariseth, the same art must be used to allay it as is before exprest.

14. If the *Pustles* go in and a flux of the belly follows (for else there is no such danger) then *Cordials* are to be used, yet moderate and not too often for fear of new *Ebullition.*

15. If much spitting (*Ptyalismus*) follow, you may hope all will go well, therefore by no means hinder it: Only with warm small Beer let their mouths be washed.

died of a contagious disease, at Boston, October 15, 1678, in the fifty-eighth year of his age.

16. When the *Pustles* are dryed and fallen, purge well, especially if it be in *Autumn*.

17. As soon as this disease therefore appears by its signs, let the sick abstein from Flesh and Wine, and open Air, let him use small Beer warmed with a Tost for his ordinary drink, and moderately when he desires it. For food use *water-gruel, water-pottage* and other things having no manifest hot quality, easy of digestion, boild Apples, and milk sometimes for change, but the coldness taken off. Let the use of his bed be according to the season of the year, and the multitude of the *Pocks*, or as sound persons are wont. In Summer let him rise according to custome, yet so as to be defended both from heat and cold in Excess, the disease will be the sooner over and less troublesome for being kept in bed nourisheth the Feaverish heat and makes the *Pocks* break out with painful inflamation.

19. In a colder season, and breaking forth of a multitude of *Pustules*, forcing the sick to keep his bed, let him be covered according to his custome in health, a moderate fire in the winter being kindled in his Chamber, morning and Evening: neither need he keep his Arms alwayes in bed, or ly still in the same place, for fear least he should sweat which is very dangerous especially to youth.

20. Before the fourth day use no medicines to drive out, nor be too strict with the sick; for by how much the more gently the *Pustules* do grow, by so much the fuller and perfecter will the Separation be.

21. On the fourth day a gentle *Cordial* may help once given.

22. From that time a small draught of warm milk (not hot) a little dy'd with *Saffron* may be given morning and evening till the *Pustules* are come to their due greatness and ripeness.

23. When the *Pustules* begin to dry and crust, least the rotten vapours strike inward, which sometimes causeth sudden death; Take morning and evening some temperate *Cordial* as four or five spoonfuls of *Malago Wine* tinged with a little *Saffron*.

24. When the *Pustules* are dryd and fallen off, purge once and again, especially in the *Autumn Pocks*.

25. Beware of anointing with *Oils, Fatts, Ointments*, and such defensives, for keeping the corrupted matter in the *Pustules* from drying up; by the moisture, they fret deeper into the Flesh, and so make the more deep Scarrs.

26. The young and lively men that are brought to a plentiful sweat in this sickness, about the eighth day the sweat stops of it self, by no means afterwards to be drawn out again; the sick thereupon feels most troublesome disrest and anguish, and then makes abundance of water and so dyes. Few young men and strong thus handled escape, except they fall into abundance of spitting or plentiful bleeding at the nose.

27. Signs discovering the Assault at first are beating pain in the head, Forehead, and temples, pain in the back, great sleepiness, glistring of the eyes, shining glimmerings seem before them, itching of them also, with tears flowing of themselves, itching of the Nose, short breath, dry Cough, oft neezing, hoarseness, heat, redness, and sense of pricking over the whole body, terrors in the sleep, sorrow and restlessness, beating of the heart, *Urine* sometimes as in health, sometime filthy from great *Ebullition*, and all this or many of these with a Feaverish distemper.

28. Signs warning of the probable Event. If they break forth easily, quickly, and soon come to ripening, if the Symptoms be gentle, the Feaver mild, and after the breaking forth it abate; If the voice be free, and breathing easie; especially if the Pox be red white, distinct, soft, few, round, sharp top'd, only without and not in the inward parts; if there be large bleeding at the nose. These signs are hopeful.

29. But such signs are doubtful, when they difficultly appear, when they sink in again, when they are black, blewish, green, hard, all in one, if the Feaver abate not with their breaking forth, if there be Swooning, difficulty of breathing, great thirst, quinsey, great unquietness, and it is very dangerous, if there be ioyn'd with it some other malignant Feaver, called by some the pestilential Pox: the *Spotted Feaver* is oft joyned with it.

30 Deadly Signs if the *Flux* of the *Belly* happen, when they are broke forth, if the Urine be bloody, or black, or the *Ordure* of that Colour; Or if pure blood be cast out by the Belly or Gumms: These Signs are for the most part deadly.

These things have I written Candid Reader, *not to inform the* Learned *Physician that hath much more cause to understand what pertains to this disease than I, but to give some light to those that have not such advantages, leaving the difficulty of this disease to the* Physicians Art, wisdome, *and* Faithfulness: *for the right managing of them in the whole Course of the disease tends both to the* Patients *safety, and the* Physicians *desired Success in his* Administrations: *For in vain is the* Physicians Art *imployed if they are not under a* Regular Regiment. *I am, though no* Physitian, *yet a well wisher to the sick: And therefore intreating the Lord to turn our hearts, and stay his hand, I am*

A Friend, Reader to thy
Welfare,
THOMAS THACHER.

2, 11. 167⅓

BOSTON, Printed and sold by *John Foster*, 1677.

The minister of Melton, about 1672, was Peter Thatcher, a man of considerable skill in medicine. He was born at Salem in 1651 and graduated from Harvard in 1671. Tradition says that he expended a considerable portion of his annual salary in procuring medicines for the sick poor. He died December 27, 1727.

In 1669 Henry Taylor, surgeon, of Boston, had his rate omitted in consideration of his agreement to attend to the sick poor.

In 1671 Dr. Samuel Stone agreed to attend to "the town's poor for twenty shillings in money and a remittance of taxes."

Several physicians of the name of Clarke resided and practiced in Boston and vicinity about this period.

Dr. Thomas Oaks, a Harvard alumnus of 1662, and William Hughes practiced medicine in Boston between 1685 and 1695. The former, a very pious man, was chosen a representative in 1689 and died in 1719, aged 75 years.

Elisha Cooke, who was born September 16, 1637, and graduated at Harvard in 1657, was a popular physician and politician. He was one of the counselors of Massachusetts in 1690 and married a daughter of Governor Leveritt. He died in 1715, in the seventy-eighth year of his age. His son, bearing the same name, succeeded him in practice, but died in 1737.

The above-mentioned and other physicians devoted themselves to medicine in Massachusetts and adjoining provinces before the close of the seventeenth century.

MEDICAL PIONEERS IN MASSACHUSETTS—EIGHTEENTH CENTURY.

Early in the eighteenth century, Dr. Nathaniel Williams, a graduate from Harvard in 1693, combined the professions of medicine and theology. His death occurred in 1739. He published in 1721 a pamphlet on the inoculation of the small-pox.

Dr. Zabdiel Boylston, son of Dr. Thomas Boylston, of Brookline, was born in Massachusetts in 1684 and died in 1766, after a long and honorable professional career. He introduced the practice of inoculation into America in 1721, meeting at first with great and violent opposition, which he was able eventually by prudence and perseverance to overcome. He published, in 1726, a historical account of inoculation in Boston. He also made communications to the Royal Society, of which he was a member.

William Douglass, M. D., a native of Scotland, was educated at Leyden and Paris as a physician and immigrated in 1718 to Boston, where he died, October 21, 1752. He was an author of some ability. He was extremely hostile to the practice of inoculation and opposed it through the public press and by a pamphlet published in 1722 and an essay on small-pox in 1730. He published, besides, an essay on epidemic fever in 1736 and in 1749 and 1755 a work entitled The British Settlements in North America, in two volumes.

Drs. Lawrence Dalhounde and Joseph Marion were practicing in Boston at the same period, and were supporters of Dr. Douglass, and also opposed the practice of inoculation, and made a sworn deposition of their personal experience of its dangerous character.

Drs. Isaac Rand, Samuel Gelston of Nantucket, and William Aspinwall, M. D., were leaders in inoculation in Massachusetts when small-pox was repeatedly epidemic. The first-named died June 19, 1749, aged 63 years. He was a native of Charlestown and a student of Dr. Thomas Graves, of that place. The last-mentioned, a native of Brookline, graduated at Harvard in 1764, and, having studied medicine with Dr. Benjamin Gale, of Connecticut, completed his medical education at Philadelphia, where he obtained the degree of M. B., in 1768. He was a surgeon in the Continental Army and one of the most prominent medical men of his time in America. He was distinguished for his success in treating small-pox and maintained for many years a private hospital near Boston for the inoculation of the same. He promptly abandoned this practice on the introduction of vaccination, which was thoroughly tested by him in his own hospital.

John Cutler was a physician of eminence during the early part of the century and was the preceptor of many medical men who rose to eminence.

Sylvester Gardiner, a native of Kingston, R. I., enjoyed the reputation of a good physician and surgeon. He was the proprietor of a large apothecary-store in Boston. He died in 1786, aged 68 years.

Benjamin Church, who graduated at Harvard College in 1754, and subsequently studied medicine with Dr. Pynchon, was popular as a physician and a man of learning and was appointed first surgeon-general of the Continental Army, but was dismissed and imprisoned for some treasonable correspondence. After languishing in prison for a year, he obtained permission to go to the West Indies; but the vessel in which he sailed was never heard of again.

Dr. James Lloyd, a native of Long Island, died in Boston, in 1810, aged 82 years. He received his medical education in Europe and was held in high esteem for his medical skill.

Drs. Thomas Bulfinch, father and son, were physicians of large business in Boston towards the close of the eighteenth century.

Dr. Miles Wentworth attended many of the wounded patriots during the siege of Boston.

Dr. Nathaniel Perkins practiced in Boston prior to the Revolution.

Drs. William Lee Perkins, M. Whitworth, Lord, John Perkins, Philip Godfrey, Roberts, Barret, Charles Pynchon, and Benjamin Curtis, all practiced medicine in Boston about the year 1764 and were in good repute. The last-named graduated at Harvard, and after leaving college studied medicine with Dr. Joseph Gardiner and settled in Boston, maintaining a good reputation and practice until his death, which occurred in 1784, in the thirty-second year of his age.

Joseph Gardiner was held in high esteem as a physician and surgeon, and, although well-informed, affected to despise book-learning. He died in 1788.

Joseph Whipple, a student of the preceding, was a practitioner of note and for some time secretary of the Massachusetts Medical Society. He acquired a large professional business in Boston, where he resided. His death occurred in 1804, in the forty-eighth year of his age.

Drs. Nathaniel Walker Appleton and Charles Jarvis, of Boston, were contemporaries. Dr. Appleton graduated at Harvard, and in 1773 began the study of medicine with Dr. Holyoke, of Salem. Dr. Jarvis, son of Colonel Jarvis, having graduated at Harvard in 1766, went to Europe to complete his education. After his return he settled in Boston as a physician. He was a zealous patriot and took an active part in the struggle for independence, being a member of the legislature and a surgeon in the Army. He died, November 15, 1807, while surgeon of the marine hospital at Charlestown. His wife was a granddaughter of the first Baron Pepperille.

John Sprague, having graduated at Harvard in 1737, became the pupil of Dr. Dalhounde, of Boston, whose daughter he subsequently married. He had an extensive practice and was sent to the convention for framing a State-constitution, in 1779. He died in 1789, aged 90 years.

John Homans, having served his country throughout the Revolution as a surgeon, settled to the practice of medicine in Boston.

Passing to other towns, we meet with Dr. John Pope, who early resided in Stoughton, where he practiced medicine, exacting no fee for professional services rendered on the Sabbath. Died in Boston in 1796, aged 55.

Thomas Little practiced in Plymouth from 1700 to 1712, the year of his death.

Joseph Richards was born at Dedham, April 18, 1701, and graduated from Harvard in 1721. He studied medicine and practiced in his native town. He served as a military officer, and was a magistrate at the time of his death, February 28, 1761, being then 59 years of age.

Elijah Danforth graduated from Harvard College in 1703 and, having studied medicine, commenced practice in Roxbury, but removed to Dorchester some years previous to his death, which occurred in 1753. He had accumulated a handsome fortune as the result of his professional labors.

The second regularly-educated physician of Scituate, Benjamin Stockbridge, was born in that town in 1704. He was a student of Dr. Bulfinch, of Boston, and himself educated many young men for the profession. His practice extended over all the old colony and was considerable in Worcester and Ipswich.

John Corbett was the earliest physician of Bellingham. His son John also practiced very successfully in the same town. In the latter part of his life his powers of speech and locomotion failed; yet, with a chair on wheels and a well-trained horse, he continued to attend a large circle of patients until near his death, which occurred in 1794.

Nathaniel Ames was born at Bridgewater, July 22, 1708, practiced medicine in Dedham, and died at Dorchester, July 11, 1764, at the age of 56 years. Having acquired a local fame in the science of astronomy, he published an almanac annually from 1735 to the time of his death.

Upon the death of Dr. Elijah Danforth, in 1736, William Holden succeeded to his practice in Dorchester and vicinity. Dr. Holden was born at Cambridge, March 4, 1713, and died in Dorchester, March 30, 1776.

Benjamin Richards was born at Weymouth in 1714, and died in 1755. He practiced medicine in his native town, sustained a good professional reputation, and enjoyed an extensive practice until his death.

Henry Turner died at Quincy, January 21, 1773, aged 84 years. He was a native of England, and was educated in London as an apothecary, immigrated to Massachusetts as early as 1715, but never acquired an extensive practice. His son, bearing the same name, was a regularly-educated physician and practiced in Quincy until his death, which occurred previous to that of his father.

The earliest physician of Dorchester Village, (now Canton,) which was organized in 1717, was Dr. Belcher. Tradition says of the doctor that he was no inconsiderable athlete, and that he and his minister, the latter also a mighty wrestler, unwilling to compromise the dignity of their respective callings by a public trial of strength, often retired alone to the forest to renew the sports of their youth.

Dr. Jonathan Thayer, a successful physician of Bellingham, died in 1760, in the forty-third year of his age.

Isaac Otis, a gentleman of uncommon accomplishments, was the first resident physician of Scituate who was regularly educated for the profession. He died in 1718.

Dr. Daniel Rogers, son of Dr. John Rogers, perished in a snow-storm, while visiting a patient on Hampton Beach, December 1, 1722.

James Jerauld, a native of France, settled at Medfield about the year 1733, where he owned a large estate, which he cultivated by slave-labor. He practiced medicine successfully for many years, and died October 17, 1760, leaving his professional practice to his nephew and adopted son, James Jerauld, who also became eminent as a medical man. The latter died March 28, 1802, aged 80. He was elected a member of the convention for framing a State-constitution.

Dr. Ammi Cutter, a native of Yarmouth, Me., graduated at Harvard, 1752. He studied medicine with Dr. Clement Jackson, in Portsmouth, was appointed and served as surgeon to the New Hampshire troops in 1758. At the commencement of the Revolution he was commissioned surgeon and was appointed physician-general of the eastern department, and always acquitted himself with credit. He died in 1820, aged 85.

Dr. Ezra Dean, believed to have been the first physician that settled in Taunton, Mass., practiced there for many years. He died in 1737.

Dr. William Dexter studied medicine with Dr. Edward Flint, of Shrewsbury. He was commissioned in 1775 and was in the battle of Bunker Hill. He died December 4, 1785.

Joseph Baxter, son of the Rev. Joseph Baxter, second minister of Medfield, graduated from Harvard in 1724 and studied and practiced medicine. He died of small-pox, in 1745.

John Wilson, the first resident physician of Braintree, (now Quincy,) enjoyed an excellent reputation and practiced until his death, in 1727. He probably finished his medical education in London. His father, the Rev. John Wilson, was also a physician.

Ebenezer Doggett, the first resident physician of Walpole, died, February 26, 1782, of cancer of the breast. His professional visits often extended to Foxboro' and Wrentham.

Edward Stedman succeeded to the medical practice of Dr. John Wilson, who died at Braintree in 1727.

William Whiting, of Great Barrington, an eminent physician, was a native of Norwich, Conn., where he studied medicine with Dr. John Bulkley. He settled at Great Barrington about 1760 and held the reputation of being the best physician in that section. He was respectively judge of the common-pleas court, member of the Provincial Congress, and delegate to the convention for framing the State-constitution in 1779. He died of dropsy, December 8, 1792, aged 63 years.

Cotton Tufts was born at Medford in May, 1731, and graduated from Harvard in 1749. He studied medicine with his brother, Dr. Simon Tufts, of Medford, and settled in Weymouth, where he enjoyed a reputation for professional ability and had a very large practice. He was a member of the convention that adopted the Constitution of the United States, served as a member of the State-senate for a number of years, and was president of the Massachusetts Medical Society from 1787 to 1793. He died December 8, 1815.

Oliver Prescott, a physician of Hanover, had conferred upon him, in 1792, the degree of M. D., *pro honoris causa*, by Harvard. He was born April 27, 1731, graduated from Harvard in 1750, and received the degree of A. M. in 1753. He was town-clerk 13 and selectman 32 years. He held respectively the offices of major, lieutenant-colonel, colonel, and brigadier-general, previous to the Revolution. He was a justice throughout the Commonwealth, a member of the board of war, and a member of the council of the State, and in 1779 was appointed judge of probate for Middlesex County, which latter office he retained during life. In 1778 he was appointed third major-general in the Continental Army and in 1781 second major-general, but resigned soon after on account of sickness. He died November 4, 1804.

His son, Oliver Prescott, jr., was also a prominent physician. He entered Harvard in 1779, and the degrees of A. B. and A. M. were conferred upon him in due course. Having studied medicine with his father and Dr. Lloyd of Boston, he settled in Groton, and soon acquired an extensive practice, not only in that place, but in several other towns in the vicinity. He was appointed a surgeon in General Lincoln's army, raised in 1787, to suppress Shay's rebellion. He occupied the respective offices of town-clerk, chairman of the selectmen, justice of the peace, and representative of the town in the General Court in 1810. His reputation as a physician was even greater than that of his father, though he was never so popular as a man.

Giles Crouch Kellogg, a native of Hadley, was the adopted son of Dr. Crouch, an excellent but eccentric physician of Hadley, who came originally from England. He graduated from Harvard in 1751, studied medicine, and acquired a reputation for proficiency in his profession. His name appears in the charter of the Massachusetts Medical Society. He died about 1787, at the age of 54 years.

Charles Stockbridge, son of Dr. Benjamin Stockbridge, was born at Scituate in the year 1734, graduated from Harvard in 1754, and pursued the study of medicine under his father. He was a skillful physician, a gentleman of pleasing manners, and accomplished in literature. Died in 1806, aged 72 years.

John Metcalf was born at Wrentham, July 3, 1734, and studied medicine with Dr. Joseph Hewes, of Providence, R. I. Commenced practice in Franklin in 1758, but abandoned it in 1808, owing to old age and infirmities. He removed to St. Albans, Vt., where he died August 22, 1822, aged 88 years.

Joseph Jacobs, of Scituate, was a man of talent and a skillful and successful physician. He was one of the proprietors of the Jacobs Mills, and a large landholder in Scituate and Hanover. He married Mary, daughter of Edward Dorchester, about 1734.

Micajah Sawyer, M. D., son of Dr. Enoch Sawyer, a physician of Newburyport, was born July 15, 1737, and graduated from Harvard in 1756. He studied medicine with his father, and began the practice of his profession in his native town, and soon acquired a great reputation as a physician, and received the honorary degree of M. D. from Harvard. When the committee of safety and correspondence was organized in 1776, he was made a member, and was conspicuous as a patriot throughout the whole period of the Revolution. He was enrolled in various literary and benevolent societies and died September 29, 1815.

The town-clerk of Stoughton, Dr. George Crossman, maintained during life a good reputation as a physician. He died at Canton, September 25, 1805, at the age of 68 years.

John Druce, a native of Brookline, graduated from Harvard in 1738 and studied medicine at Watertown. He settled as a physician at Wrentham, about the year 1740, but died of consumption at the age of 55 years.

Dr. Samuel Leslie Scammell emigrated from England in 1738 and settled in that part of Mendon now called Milford, and there practiced medicine until his death, in 1752. He was 45 years of age. His son, bearing the same name, was also a practitioner of medicine and was the father of Colonel Alexander Scammell, a distinguished officer of the American revolutionary army, and Dr. John Scammell, a physician of considerable celebrity. The son of the last-mentioned, Dr. John Scammell, was born at Milford, in 1761, and studied medicine with his father. On the death of his maternal grandfather, Dr. John Corbett, he removed to Bellingham, to take possession of the estate and practice bequeathed him by the doctor. He served for a short period in the Continental Army. About a year previous to his death he fractured his thigh, which never re-united. He died, March 9, 1845, at the age of 84 years.

Samuel Holten was born at Salem Village, (now Danvers,) June 19, 1738, studied medicine with Dr. Jonathan Prince, and settled in Gloucester to practice his profession, but shortly after removed to his native town. In 1775 he espoused the cause of the patriots, and was placed upon several important committees of the Continental Congress, of which body he was a member. He was also on the medical board for the examination of applicants for appointment to the medical department of the Army. In 1777 he was one of the delegates from Massachusetts who assisted in framing the Articles of Confederation of the United Colonies, and later was chosen delegate to the American Congress, and affixed his ratifying signature to the Constitution of the United States. He was afterward elected president of that body. In 1796 he was appointed judge of the probate court of Essex County, which office he resigned in 1815, after having been in public station over forty-seven years. With a majestic form, a graceful person, and engaging manners, he was eminently popular. He died, January 2, 1816, in the seventy-eighth year of his age.

Jonathan Davis, a native of Maine, graduated from Harvard in 1738, and was for years a reputable physician in Roxbury; he died in 1801.

Dr. James Baker was born September 5, 1739, at Dorchester, and graduated from Harvard in 1760; studied theology and became a preacher, but subsequently turned his attention to medicine, which, after practicing a few years, he relinquished, about the year 1780, for other pursuits.

William Baylies, a native of Uxbridge, an eminent physician of Massachusetts, graduated from Harvard in 1760, established himself at Dighton, and became very successful and popular in the practice of medicine. He was a member of the American Academy of Arts and Sciences, of the Massachusetts Medical Society, and of the Massachusetts Historical Society. He represented Dighton in the legislature of the State, occupied a seat in three Provincial Congresses and in the State-convention that adopted the Federal Constitution, and was a judge of the court of common pleas and register of probate for Bristol County.

In 1800 he was one of the presidential electors; and, after a long and useful life, died, June 17, 1826, at the age of 86.

Aaron Wright, of Medway, was born in 1742 and studied medicine with Dr. Thomas Kittridge, whose daughter he subsequently married. Upon the completion of his studies he commenced practice, but the amputation of one of his legs was rendered necessary by disease, notwithstanding which misfortune we find him, in connection with Dr. Jerauld, conducting a small-pox-hospital in Medfield, about 1780.

Dr. Elisha Savil graduated from Harvard in 1743. His reputation as a physician was good, and he acquired an extensive practice, not only in Quincy, where he resided, but also in Milton and the middle and south precincts of Braintree. He died of lung-fever, April 30, 1768, in his forty-fourth year.

Isaac Rand, son of Dr. Isaac Rand, of Charlestown, who died in 1790, aged 71, was born April 27, 1743, graduated from Harvard in 1761, studied medicine with Dr. Lloyd and his father, and settled to practice in Boston in 1764. He was very proficient in the exact sciences, and was appointed, with Samuel Williams, (afterward professor of natural philosophy at Harvard,) to accompany Prof. Winthrop to Newfoundland, to observe the transit of Venus in 1761. He was eminent in his profession and wrote several medical essays and treatises. He died, September 11, 1822, in the eightieth year of his age.

James Pecker, son of Dr. James Pecker, of Haverhill, graduated from Harvard, studied medicine, and settled in Boston. He stood high as a professional man and was the first vice-president of the Massachusetts Medical Society. Towards the close of life he was afflicted with stone in his bladder, which was successfully removed by Dr. Rand. He died, in the year 1794, in the seventieth year of his age.

Gad Hitchcock, D. D., who served as minister of Pembroke fifty-five years, was also a practitioner of medicine. He graduated from Harvard in the year 1743 and died, August 8, 1803, at the age of 85 years.

Dr. Seth Ames, son of Dr. Nathaniel Ames, of Dedham, was born in 1743 and graduated from Harvard in 1764. He served as surgeon of Colonel Read's regiment in the Continental Army and located at Amherst, N. H., but his failing health obliged him to return to his native town, where he died, January 1, 1778.

Ebenezer Hunt was born at Northampton in 1744, graduated from Harvard in 1764, and, having studied medicine with Dr. Charles Pynchon, of Springfield, settled to practice in his native town in 1768. He had an extensive practice; and it is said that he possessed an unusual sagacity in discerning the nature of diseases. He was, for a considerable period, a member of the legislature and for four years occupied a seat in the State-senate.

Dr. Ephraim Wales, a native of Randolph, graduated from Harvard in 1768, and studied medicine with Dr. Amos Putnam, of Danvers. In

1770 he settled in his native parish, acquired a large practice, and instructed numerous pupils. He died, April 7, 1805, aged 59 years.

Phineas Holden, son of Dr. William Holden, was born at Dorchester, January 31, 1744, and, having studied medicine with his father, practiced in the town of his nativity until his death, 1819. In 1792, by vote of the town-council, he was permitted to build a small-pox-hospital on Dorchester Neck.

The first resident physician of Stoughton was Nathan Bucknam, who practiced there subsequently to 1744. He was probably the son of Rev. Nathan Bucknam, of Medway.

Enos Sumner was born in Milton in 1746 and practiced medicine there from 1768 till his death, June 8, 1796.

Samuel Gardner, son of the Rev. John Gardner, of Stow, graduated from Harvard in 1746 and practiced medicine in Milton from 1753 till his death, in 1777.

Elijah Hewins was born in 1747, and studied medicine with Dr. Young, of Boston. He afterward served as a surgeon in the Continental Army. At the close of the war he removed to Sharon, and for twenty years held an extensive practice in Foxboro' and Walpole, as well as Sharon. A few years previous to his death he was stricken with paralysis, which obliged him to relinquish his professional duties. He died in 1827, aged 80 years.

Lemuel Hewins was a student of Dr. Nathaniel White, whose daughter he married. He settled at Sharon, which was incorporated in 1765, and was, probably, the first physician of that borough. At the commencement of his professional career he enjoyed a considerable practice, but, his habits being unfavorable to success, his business soon declined.

Dr. Jeremiah Hall was born in Scituate, December 22, 1748, and settled at Pembroke in 1764. He attained the reputation of an excellent physician and in 1775 was a member of the Provisional Congress.

Lemuel Hayward was born at Braintree, March 22, 1749, and graduated from Harvard in the year 1768. For one year after his graduation he taught the public school at Milton and subsequently commenced the study of medicine under Dr. Joseph Warren. Having completed his studies, by the advice of his preceptor he settled at Jamaica Plains, where he acquired a large and lucrative practice. In 1775 he was appointed a hospital-surgeon by Congress, but resigned his commission on the removal of the Army southward. In 1783 he removed to Boston and in 1784 was elected member of the Massachusetts Medical Society. He died March 20, 1822.

Joseph Orne, an eminent physician of Salem and one of the original members of the Massachusetts Medical Society, was born in 1749, graduated from Harvard in 1765, and studied medicine with Dr. Holyoke. He settled in 1770 at Beverly, but removed to Salem, his native town, where he secured an enviable reputation as a physician. He died, January 28, 1786, of pulmonary consumption, at the age of 37.

Thomas Lowthrain, a native of Perth, Scotland, died at Medfield December 15, 1749. He was a practitioner of medicine of that place and was highly esteemed.

Dr. Edward Augustus Holyoke, the first president of the Massachusetts Medical Society, was the son of Rev. Augustus Holyoke, who was president of Harvard College about 1746. He studied medicine with Col. Thomas Berry, a distinguished physician of Ipswich, and in 1749 settled at Salem, where he practiced medicine nearly eighty years, until his death, which occurred March 31, 1829, at the age of 100 years.

Aaron Dexter, a distinguished physician of Boston, for many years a professor in Harvard, of which institution he was an alumnus, was born at Malden, November 11, 1750, and died, February 28, 1829, aged 79 years. He studied medicine with Dr. Samuel Danforth, of Boston, and commenced practice in the latter place about the close of the revolutionary war. In 1783 he was elected professor of chemistry and materia medica in the medical department of Harvard, which position he filled until 1816, when he was constituted emeritus-professor.

Dr. Benjamin Gott, of Marlboro', practiced medicine during the epidemic of 1749 and 1750 and rendered valuable assistance to the afflicted inhabitants. He married a daughter of Rev. Robert Breck, of Northboro'.

Thomas Kast, son of Dr. Philip Godfrist Kast, was born in Boston, August 12, 1750; graduated from Harvard in 1769 and commenced immediately the study of medicine with his father. In 1770 he was appointed surgeon's mate of the British ship Rose; but, on arriving in England in 1772, he resigned, and spent two years in attending the clinics of the hospitals of London. In 1774 he returned to Boston and commenced the practice of his profession. His professional business was large and he was reputed to be a skillful surgeon. He died June 20, 1820, in his seventieth year.

Dr. Oliver Patridge was born at Hatfield in 1751 and removed to Stockbridge in 1771. Two years later he began the active practice of his profession, which he continued until his death, in 1848.

Dr. Barnabas Binney, a surgeon in the Continental Army, was born in 1751. His father was a Boston merchant and his mother, formerly Miss Ings, was a lady of high intellectual culture. He graduated from Rhode Island College (now Brown University) in 1774, but his medical education was acquired in Philadelphia and London. In 1776 he entered the Army as hospital-physician and surgeon, which position he retained until the close of the war, and in which he distinguished himself by his professional ability. His health was so impaired by military service that he lived but a few years, his death taking place June 21, 1787, at the age of 36.

Abijah Richardson was born in Medway, August 30, 1752, and studied two years in Harvard before commencing the study of medicine. In 1776, after completing his medical education, he entered the Army as a surgeon's mate, but soon received a surgeon's commission, which he retained until the termination of hostilities. He returned to his native town and maintained a respectable practice until the time of his death, May 10, 1822, at the age of 70 years.

Dr. John Barnard Swett was born at Marblehead, June 1, 1752, and graduated from Harvard in 1767. He studied medicine at Edinburgh under the celebrated Cullen and also attended the hospitals of France and England. Having completed his medical education, he returned to America and entered the Continental Army as a surgeon. In 1780 he resigned his commission, commenced practice in Newburyport, and soon had a large and responsible business. He fell a victim to the yellow fever that prevailed in Newburyport in 1796, aged 44.

Samuel Kingsly Glover was born in Milton, in 1753, and entered Harvard College, but before the time of his graduation the Revolution commenced and study at the college was suspended. Shortly after he joined the Army as surgeon's mate, and as such, and in the capacity of surgeon to several war-vessels, he served until 1778, when he resigned his commission and returned to his native town. He did not resume full practice on his return, but devoted considerable time to a private small-pox-hospital. He died July 1, 1839, aged 86 years.

Dr. Joseph Warren, memorable for his patriotism, was in the enjoyment of a large practice and of great popular esteem before the battle of Bunker Hill, in which his life was sacrificed. His life has been so frequently and faithfully sketched that an extended notice here is uncalled for.

John Warren, M. D., brother of General Joseph Warren, was born, at Roxbury, July 28, 1753. He subsequently studied medicine, commenced practice at Salem, and acted as surgeon at the battle of Lexington. Hastening to Boston on the report that a battle had been fought there, he learned that his brother had perished in it, and immediately offered his own services to his country. Though only 22 years old, he was appointed senior surgeon of the hospital at Cambridge, accompanied the Army in its two subsequent campaigns, and in 1777 became surgeon-in-chief of the military hospitals at Boston, which position he retained until the close of the war. In 1780 he gave to a class of medical students a course of dissections and in 1783 was made professor of anatomy and surgery in the medical school of Harvard University. He died of inflammation of the lungs, April 4, 1815, at the age of 61 years.

William Eustis, M. D., a surgeon in the Continental Army, was born, at Cambridge, June 10, 1753, and, having graduated from Harvard in 1772, immediately commenced the study of medicine with Dr. Joseph Warren. At the commencement of the Revolution, he entered the Army as a surgeon of a regiment in the field, but in 1775 was appointed hospital-surgeon, and at the close of the war resumed his practice in Boston. In 1800 he was elected member of Congress and in 1809 was appointed

Secretary of War by the President, (Mr. Madison,) which position he resigned after the surrender of General Hull. He was delegated embassador to Holland, and upon his return in 1821 was again sent to Congress, and for four consecutive terms occupied a seat in that body. In 1823 he was elected governor, and died in Boston, February 6, 1825, at the age of 72 years.

James Thacher, M. D., was born in 1754, entered the Army as a surgeon's mate in 1775, and was promoted to a surgeoncy in the following year. He was present at many battles, but after the surrender of Yorktown retired from the military service. He received the degree of A. M. from Harvard and M. D. from both Harvard and Dartmouth; was a distinguished antiquarian, as well as a miscellaneous and medical writer. Died at Plymouth, May 24, 1844, at the age of 90 years.

Dr. Amos Holbrook, a prominent physician of Milton, was born at Bellingham in 1754; served in the Continental Army as surgeon's mate, and subsequently spent some time in the hospitals of Paris, adding to his store of professional knowledge. His practice was very extensive, and not only did he engross the chief medical business of Milton, but also of Dorchester. He died June 17, 1842, aged 88 years.

Dr. Cornelius Kollock, whose death occurred January 22, 1754, was the second resident physician of Wrentham.

Dr. Moses Baker, a Friend, and it is supposed a fellow-pupil of the celebrated Dr. Benjamin Church, of Boston, settled in the south precinct of Braintree (now Randolph) in 1755. He had considerable practice in the parish in which he resided, as well as the neighboring ones. His death occurred December 10, 1781.

Dr. Shirley Erving, the grandson of Governor William Shirley, entered Harvard College, where he pursued his studies some years, but did not graduate. He studied medicine, located at Portland, and became eminent in his profession. Towards the close of life he relinquished the active duties of his calling and removed to Boston, where he died July 8, 1813, at the age of 55.

Dr. Samuel Danforth, of Cambridge, graduated from Harvard in 1758 and studied medicine with Dr. Isaac Rand, of Boston. When the revolutionary war broke out, he was judge of probate for Middlesex County; subsequently resided in Weston and in Newport, R. I., and finally settled permanently in Boston. His death, which occurred November 16, 1827, in the eighty-seventh year of his age—after sixty years' devotion to the wants of the sick—was caused by a paralytic affection.

Josiah Bartlett, M. D., was born in Charlestown in 1759 and died, March 5, 1820, of apoplexy. He studied medicine with Dr. Israel Foster, surgeon in charge of the Boston military hospital, and upon completing his studies entered the Army as Dr. Foster's assistant, and served as such until the end of the year 1780. He also served at different times as surgeon to two war-vessels. Upon the termination of the war, he resumed the practice of his profession in Charlestown. He wrote several medical and miscellaneous works, among which The Progress of Medical Science in Massachusetts and The History of Charlestown are the best known.

Dr. Joseph Le Baron, of Plymouth, probably the son of Dr. Francis Le Baron, previously mentioned, practiced medicine in that town until his death, which occurred in 1761; Dr. Lazarus Le Baron also practiced there from 1720 to 1773, and Dr. Lazarus Le Baron, jr., till 1784.

Drs. Thomas Swain and Eben Harden Goss practiced medicine in Ipswich about the year 1771.

Thomas Welch, a surgeon in the Continental Army, was born in 1751, and graduated from Harvard in 1772. After the war he enjoyed an extensive practice in Boston; was attached to the marine hospital, and at a later period was appointed quarantine-physician of the port. At the time of his death, which happened in February, 1831, in the eightieth year of his age, he was the oldest member of the Boston Medical Faculty and the only survivor of the original founders of the Massachusetts Medical Society.

Daniel Fisher, of Wrentham, who died March 29, 1774, was a practitioner of medicine in that place.

Timothy Child, M. D., was born at Deerfield, of English parents. Having spent some time at Harvard College, he studied medicine with Dr. Williams and commenced practice at Pittsfield in 1771. Immediately after the battle of Lexington he was appointed surgeon of Colonel Patterson's regiment, but shortly after resigned his commission and, returning home, resumed his professional business. He died in 1821, at the age of 73 years. He was called several times during life to fill the positions of representative and senator in the State legislature.

Dr. Prince practiced medicine at Salem during the revolutionary war.

James Mann, M. D., a native of Wrentham, graduated in 1776 from Harvard and received the honorary degree of M. D. from Brown University in 1815. After leaving Harvard he began the study of medicine under Dr. Danforth, of Boston, and, having completed his studies, immediately joined the Continental Army as a surgeon, but after three years' service his enfeebled health compelled him to resign. In 1812 Dr. Mann was appointed hospital-surgeon in the United States Army and during the war that followed was attached to the medical staff on the northern frontier. In 1816 he published a volume of medical sketches of the war of 1812. He died in New York in November, 1832, aged 70.

Dr. Marsh, formerly of Hingham, practiced in Hanover about the year 1780.

Jabez Fuller, a practitioner of medicine, died at Medfield, October 5, 1781.

Peter Hobart, of Hingham, removed to Hanover about the year 1783, and there resided and practiced until his death, in 1793.

Nathaniel Breed resided in Ipswich, as physician, from 1786 to 1789 and took some part in the town-affairs.

Dr. William Thomas, a practitioner of medicine, resided in Plymouth until his death, which occurred in 1802.

John Frunk, one of the most distinguished physicians of Rutland, died in 1807. He was one of the founders of the Massachusetts Medical Society.

Dr. Brooks practiced medicine at Medford prior to the year 1773.

MASSACHUSETTS SURGEONS IN THE REVOLUTIONARY WAR.

The following-named physicians of Massachusetts served on the medical staff of the American Army during the revolutionary war : Henry Adams, Samuel Adams, Eben Ballentine, Origen Bringham, Ezekiel Brown, Abijah Cheever, John Crane, Lemuel Cushing of Hanover, John Duffield, Samuel Finley, Joseph Fisk, Isaac G. Graham, William Loughton, Benjamin Morgan, Thaddeus Thompson, Samuel Whitewell, Daniel Shute, James B. E. Finley, John Thomas, and William Laughlin.

Surgeon Daniel Bartlett died in Worcester County, Mass., December 25, 1819 ; William Coggeswell died January 1, 1831, in Rockingham County, N. H.

Francis Le Baron Goodwin served until the close of the war, in Colonel Henry Jackson's regiment, as surgeon.

Walter Hastings entered the medical department of the Army early in 1775.

Thomas Kittredge was commissioned surgeon of Colonel James Frye's regiment from Essex, May 2, 1775.

Surgeon Percival Hall died September 25, 1825.

Surgeon John Lynn, of Boston, was originally from Pennsylvania, and leaving the Army after the cessation of hostilities returned to his native State, where he died about the year 1792, in the forty-third year of his age.

Surgeon David Townsend died in Suffolk County, Mass., April 13, 1829.

MISCELLANEA RESPECTING EARLY MEDICAL PRACTICE.

Governor John Winthrop, the civil head of the Massachusetts colony, although bred to the law, is said to have been skilled in practice of medicine, distributing as charity Van Helmont's remedies. His son John, the first governor of Connecticut, and a Dublin graduate, was a physician of ability, and a record of cases treated by him, it is said, still exists in manuscript. He was also one of the founders of the Royal Society of England, being in London at the time of its organization, and made to it several communications. He died in 1671, aged 71 years. [1]

Many other names might be added to this extensive list, but those

---
[1] Douglass's Summary, p. 428.

given are quite sufficient to show how numerous and influential was the medical practitioner in colonial times.

The colony of Massachusetts passed a law in 1649, forbidding chirurgeons, midwives, physicians, and others to exercise or put forth any act contrary to the known rules of their respective arts, &c., the subject-matter of which was repeated in 1665 in a law enacted in the Duke of York's grant.[1]

A number of the clergymen who came to America at an early period were also educated as physicians, both in the Dutch and English

---

[1] *Chirurgions, Midwives, Physitians.*—Forasmuch as the law of God allowes no man to impaire the life or limbs of any person, but in a judicial way: It is therefore ordered, That no person or persons whatsoever imployed at any time about the bodyes of men, women, or children for preservation of life or health as chirurgions, midwives, physitians, or others, presume to exercise or put forth any act contrary to the known approved Rules of Art in each Mystery and occupation, nor exercise any force, violence, or cruelty, upon or towards the body of any; whether young or old, (no, not in the most difficult and desperate cases,) without the advice and consent of such as are skillfull in the same art, (if such may be had,) or at least of some of the wisest and gravest then present, and consent of the patient or patients if they be *mentis compotes*, much less contrary to such advice and consent, upon such severe punishment as the nature of the fact may deserve; which law, nevertheless, is not intended to discourage any from all lawfull use of their skill, but rather to incourage and direct them in the right use thereof, and inhibit and restreine the presumptuous arrogancy of such as through presidence of their own skill, or any other sinister respects, dare boldly attempt to exercise any violence upon or towards the bodyes of young or old, one or other, to the prejudice or hazard of life or limbe of man, woman, or child. [1649.]—(Ancient Charters and Laws of Massachusetts Bay, pp. 76-77; also Laws of Mass., edition of 1672, printed at Cambridge, page 28.)

The following general laws, relating to medical men and medical matters, were enacted in Massachusetts during the colonial period: An act requiring chirurgeons, midwives, and physicians to use no force or violence in their respective callings, without the consent of adepts in the same art, enacted 1649, Stat. Mass., ed. 1672, p. 28; An act to better prevent the spreading of infectious sickness, Stat. Mass., ed. 1699, p. 149; An act authorizing the selectmen to provide for those sick with contagious diseases, to prevent infection, enacted 1701, Stat. Mass., ed. 1714, p. 167; An act providing at the charge of the province a convenient house on the island called Spectacle Island, for the reception of such as shall be visited with contagious diseases, to keep them from infecting others, enacted 1717, Stat. Mass., ed. 1726, p. 261; An act empowering courts to adjourn and remove from towns appointed by law for holding courts, in case of sickness by the small-pox, enacted 1730, Stat. Mass., ed. 1759, p. 265; An act to prevent persons concealing the small-pox, and requiring a red cloath to be hung out in all infected places, enacted 1731, Stat. Mass., p. 472; An act to prevent the spreading of the small-pox and other infectious diseases and concealing the same, enacted 1742, Stat. Mass., 1763, p. 22; An act regulating the hospital on Rainsford Island, and further providing in case of infectious sickness, enacted 1743, Temp. Laws, Mass., p. 102; An act to regulate the importation of Germans and other passengers coming to settle in this province, providing that sufficient provisions and room be given them to prevent the contraction of diseases, enacted 1750, Stat. Mass., ed. 1759, p. 342; An act supplementary to the act regulating the hospital on Rainsford Island, providing for magistrates to order infectious vessels or persons to the province hospital, enacted 1758, Stat. Mass., 1789, p. 378; An act to incorporate certain physicians by the name of the Massachusetts Medical Society, enacted 1781, Stat. Mass., ed. 1789, p. 415.

settlements, but particularly in the New England colonies. For this double duty they made especial preparation, with a view to being true missionaries, before they embarked for the New World. In some instances, too, the schoolmaster was also the physician and surgeon of the neighborhood. In those days, when the literature of the profession was largely contained within the covers of Hippocrates and Galen, it was not difficult for a university-graduate to make himself familiar with the medical theories and practice of the times.

As early as 1690, hostilities began to manifest themselves between the English adherents in the New England colonies and the French immigrants and settlers in the Canadas, which were continued, and finally resulted in the subjugation of the French in 1763. These military expeditions and the military training given by them, with the demand they created for skilled medical officers, did something to advance and encourage the progress of medicine in the colonies. The condition of the profession is alluded to by Smith in his History of New York.[1]

It is true of all wars that they greatly advance medical science.[2] This is abundantly proved by history and experience.

EARLY MEDICAL PRACTICE IN NEW YORK.

The Dutch West India Company, by which New York was originally held, in their regulations or charter from the States-General, in 1629, entitled "Freedoms and Exemptions," in section xxvii, provided as follows: "The patrons and colonists shall, in particular, and in the speediest manner, endeavor to find ways and means whereby they may support a minister and a schoolmaster; that thus the service of God

---

[1] Few physicians amongst us are eminent for their skill. Quacks abound like locusts in Egypt, and too many have recommended themselves to a full and profitable practice and subsistence. This is the less to be wondered at, as the profession is under no kind of regulation. Loud as the call is, to our shame be it remembered, we have no law to protect the lives of the King's subjects from the malpractice of pretenders. Any man at his pleasure sets up for physician, apothecary, and chirurgeon. No candidates are either examined or licensed, or even sworn to fair practice.—(Smith's Hist. N. Y., p. 326.)

[2] The war which resulted in the conquest of Canada gave perhaps the first material improvement to the condition of medicine in America. The English army were accompanied by a highly respectable medical staff, most of whom landed in the city of New York and continued for some years in the neighboring territories, affording to many young Americans opportunities of attending the military hospitals and receiving professional instruction. The physicians and surgeons of the Anglo-American army gained the confidence of the public by their superior deportment and professional information and aroused the ambition of the colonial practitioners.

The military establishments in Massachusetts and New York after the Canadian war required medical and surgical attendants, so that the people had the benefit of their advice; in this manner a superior class of medical men was introduced into the community.—(Davis's History of Medical Education.)

and zeal for religion may not grow cool and be neglected among them; and that they do for the first procure a comforter for the sick."[1]

In 1738 the directors submitted a draught of a law to secure equal justice to all and to define the mode of conducting their business and raising revenues. Section vii provides "For the maintenance of preachers, *comforters of the sick*, schoolmasters, and similar necessary officers; each householder and inhabitant shall bear such contributions and public charge as shall hereafter be considered proper."[2]

Hermann Mynderts van de Bogaerdet came to the province in 1631 as surgeon to the ship Endragh.[3]

We find the name of William Deeping as chirurgeon to the ship William of London, in April, 1633, then trading in the Hudson.[4]

There arrived at Manhattan's, March 28, 1638, along with William Kieft, director-general of the West India Company or New Netherlands, Surgeons Gerritt Schult and Hans Kierstede.[5] The latter was well connected and continued in practice in the colony as late as 1661. He married Sarah, daughter of Annetje Jansen, who owned a farm on Manhattan Island and is said to have been a skillful midwife.

In 1647 William Hays and Peter Vreucht; from 1649 to 1652, Jacob Hendrickson Varvanger, Isaac Jansen, Jacob Mallenacy, and John Pau, some of them being surgeons on ships trading, practiced in New York.

Johannes La Montague,[6] a Huguenot gentleman of learning, was a skillful physician and a member of Kieft's council. He arrived in New York in 1637 and in 1641 was sent with an expedition of fifty men to defend Fort Good Hope. He held at different times various offices and positions of trust and always acquitted himself with credit.

Samuel Megapolensis,[7] son of the Rev. Johannes Megapolensis, who came to New York in 1642, was sent to Harvard College in 1657, afterward to the University of Utrecht, where he graduated in theology, and was licensed as a minister, receiving also the degree of M. D. On his return to New Amsterdam he was appointed collegiate church-pastor. He also through life engaged in the practice of medicine. He was one of the commissioners on the part of the Dutch to negotiate with the British the articles of capitulation of the province in 1664.

Dr. Abraham Staats came from Holland, settled at Fort Orange, and was a man of note in the colony as early as 1650. He assisted in making an important treaty with the Indians and in 1664 his house at Clav-

---

[1] History of the New Netherlands, p. 119.

[2] Documentary History of New York, vol. i, p. 77.

[3] Brodhead's History of the State of New York, pp. 419, 491.

[4] History of New Netherlands, p. 143.

[5] Brodhead's History of New York, pp. 408, 731, 748; History of New Netherlands, pp. 142, 181.

[6] Brodhead's New York, pp. 273, 279, 322, 550; History of New Netherlands, pp. 180, 185, 186, 266, 273.

[7] Brodhead's New York, pp. 643, 741.

erack was burned by the savages, his wife and two sons perishing in it.[1] His son Samuel, born in the province, was also a physician and was educated in Holland. He located in New York and soon rose to eminence. He died in 1715, much respected.

In 1658, according to the New York City Medical Register, there were but the following three surgeons in New Amsterdam : Kierstede, Vanevanger, and L'Orange.

Jacob D. Commer, as early as 1660, or earlier, was the leading surgeon of New Amsterdam, but subsequently removed to New Amstel, (New Castle, Del.)

Dr. J. Hughes was a practicing physician in the city as early as 1661.

In enumerating the names of the Dutch physicians who had from their learning, worth, and skill attained eminence in the colony prior to the English assumption of government in 1664, the names of Jan du Parck and Alexander C. Curtis[2] should not be omitted. The latter, in addition to practicing medicine, taught a Latin school. He returned to Holland about the time the English rule began.

Peter Jansen van den Bergh, Jacob L'Orange, Hermann Wessels, Samuel Megapolensis, Comelis van Dyck, (who died in 1687,) and Henry Taylor were in practice between 1658 and 1680.

Gysbert van Imbroeck, who married a daughter of Dr. La Montague, practiced his profession at Wiltwyck prior to 1663. His wife, who had been a prisoner with the Indians and escaped in that year, acted as guide in an expedition against the savages who had been her captors.

In 1664 the doctor was one of the delegates to the provincial assembly.[3]

Gerardus Beekman was a physician and politician and the son of William Beekman, a leading citizen of the early Dutch rule, who came to New Amsterdam in 1647 and held many positions of public trust. He died in 1707. The doctor was a member of Governor Lesler's council, and after his overthrow and execution Beekman was tried for treason, convicted, and sentenced to be hung, but was pardoned. He was afterward a member of the provincial council, under different governors. He died in 1724.[4]

In 1661 Michiel de Marco Cherts[5] was surgeon for the Company at New Amstel, now New Castle, Del.

Dr. Jacob von Belcamp was a druggist at New Amstel.

William Beltsnyder was paid for furnishing medicines and was probably also an apothecary or druggist.

The following-named persons were paid, it appears, as comforters of

---

[1] Brodhead's History of New York, pp. 530, 733, 748; O'Callahan's History of New Netherlands, vol. ii, p. 519.
[2] Brodhead's History of New York.
[3] Brodhead's History of New York, pp. 712, 729.
[4] Valentine's Manual of Common Council of New York, 1864, p. 567.
[5] Documentary History of New York, vol. ii, pp. 182-191.

the sick by the Company: Evart Pietersen, Arent Evertsen, and Molenaer.

In 1666 Mr. De Hinse [1] was a French physician and resident surgeon of Fort Albany.

Giles Geodineau,[2] who signed himself chirurgo-physician, was a French Huguenot and a physician of some ability. He received letters of denization in New York, August 26, 1686.

Dr. Lockhart,[3] a Scotch physician, was surgeon to the fort and practiced in Albany in 1689.

Johannes Kerfbyle,[4] a native of Holland and a graduate of Leyden, was an eminent practitioner of medicine in New York from about the period of the Dutch surrender until 1693. He was prominent as a citizen, influential in society, a member of the Reformed Church, and enjoyed a large professional business about the year 1686. In 1691 he made, by direction of the civil authorities, a post-mortem examination of the body of Governor Slaughter, which is said to be the first recorded autopsy in America. His first wife was Catharine Hug, who came to the colony with him, and upon her death he married, in 1704, Margaret Provoost. He was a member of the provincial council in 1698. He died in the city of New York.

At the time of which we are writing the midwives were licensed to practice in Holland when found qualified, and the emigrants from that country to New Amsterdam brought the same customs and practices with them to their new homes. We might give the names of many who practiced with reputation in New York. There are a number of city-ordinances referring to them.[5]

The councilors and directors of Amsterdam possessed nearly arbitrary powers as to legislative authority. Their acts were, in the main, protective of the rights of the people and they administrated equal justice

---

[1] Documentary History of New York, vol. iii, p. 127.
[2] Documentary History of New York, vol. iii, p. 716.
[3] Documentary History of New York, vol. iii, p. 618.
[4] Valentine's Manual of Common Council of New York, 1864, p. 590.
[5] *New York City ordinance, July* 16, 1716.—It is ordained that no woman within this corporation shall exercise the employment of midwife until she have taken oath before the mayor, recorder, or an alderman, (the terms of which are prescribed,) to the following effect: That she will be diligent and ready to help any woman in labor, whether poor or rich; that in time of necessity she will not forsake the poor woman and go to the rich; that she will not cause or suffer any woman to name or put any other father to the child, but only him which is the very true father thereof, indeed, according to the utmost of her power; that she will not suffer any woman to pretend to be delivered of a child who is not indeed, neither to claim any other woman's child for her own; that she will not suffer any woman's child to be murdered or hurt; and as often as she shall see any peril or jeopardy, either in the mother or child, she will call in other midwives for counsel; that she will not administer any medicine to produce miscarriage; that she will not enforce a woman to give more for her services than is right; that she will not collude to keep secret the birth of a child; will be of good behavior; will not conceal the births of bastards, &c.—(Manual of the Corporation of the City of New York, 1858, p. 564.)

to the different professions and classes remote from established courts of justice.[1]

As showing the spirit of legislation of the times in relation to medical men, the following is worthy of note. The act aimed to impose a sort of detective-duty upon the surgeon which could not be submitted to by the profession, and no doubt was a dead letter.

In December, 1657, a city-ordinance was passed by the schout,[2] burgomaster, and schepens,[3] giving notice "To all chirurgeons of the city that when they are called to dress a wound they shall ask the patient who wounded him and that information thereof be given to the schout."[4]

In the Duke of York's laws, enacted about 1665 for the government of the province of New York, when Nantucket, Martha's Vineyard, Normansland, and the Elizabeth Islands were also considered as lying within the Duke's patent, a stringent law relating to chirurgeons, midwives, and physicians was passed, which, as it may be found to possess some historical interest and is not generally available to readers, is given in full in a note.[5]

Dr. William van Rasenburgh was surgeon to the colony of New Amstel, on the Delaware, November 3, 1659, to 1662.

---

[1] *From the Dutch Records, February* 2, 1652.—" On the petition of the chirurgeons of New Amsterdam, that none but they alone be allowed to shave; the director and council understand that shaving doth not appertain exclusively to chirurgery, but is an appendix thereunto; that no man can be prevented operating on himself, nor to do another the friendly act, provided it be through courtesy, and not for gain, which is hereby forbidden. It was then further ordered that ship-barbers shall not be allowed to dress any wounds nor administer any potions on shore without the previous knowledge and special consent of the petitioners, or at least of Doctor La Montague." This, says the editor of the New York City Medical register, is the earliest order on record regulating the practice of medicine in the State.—(Medical Register, city of New York 1865, p. 198.)

[2] Sheriff.

[3] Justices.

[4] Valentine's Manual of Corporation of New York for 1858, p. 537.

[5] *Chirurgeons, Midwives, Physicians.*—That no person or persons whatever employed about the bodys of men, women, or children for the preservation of life or health as chirurgeons, midwives, physicians, or others, presume to put forth or exercise any act contrary to the known approved rule of art in each mystery or occupation, or exercise any force, violence, or cruelty upon or towards the body of any, whether young or old, without the advice and consent of such as are skilful in the same art, (if such may be had,) or at least of some of the wisest and gravest then present, and consent of the patient or patients if they be *mentis compotes*, much less contrary to such advice and consent, upon such severe punishment as the nature of the fact may deserve; which law, nevertheless, is not intended to discourage any from all lawful use of their skill, but rather to encourage and direct them in the right use thereof, and to inhibit and restrain the presumptious arrogance of such as, through confidence of their own skill or any other sinister respects, dare boldly attempt to exercise any violence upon or towards the body of young or old, one or other, to the prejudice or hazard of the life or limb of man, woman, or child.—(Picture of New York, p. 169.)

NEW YORK PHYSICIANS OF THE EIGHTEENTH CENTURY.

Naturally enough, at the beginning of the eighteenth century, owing to the increased population in the colonies, a greater number of medical men of note were found in them, many of whom, being practitioners in New York, are mentioned by Dr. Francis in his anniversary-discourse before the New York Academy of Medicine, 1847. The following are the names of a few of the more prominent physicians of that period:

Drs. Lucal van Eflinchoone was from Germany and Robert Brett and Thomas Thornbill from Great Britain.

John van Beuren was from a place of that name near Amsterdam, in Holland. He was a pupil of the celebrated Booerhaave and a graduate of Leyden. Shortly after his arrival in New York, early in 1700, he was appointed physician to the almshouse. His son, Beekman van Beuren, who was born in New York in 1727 and died in 1812, succeeded to the same position, and from this ancestral stock has sprung the numerous and respectable family of this name scattered throughout the United States.

Dr. Cadwallader Colden, born, 1688, at Dunse, in Scotland, after winning literary honors at the University of Edinburgh, in 1705, and having studied medicine, settled in Philadelphia in 1708. He practiced in Pennsylvania until the year 1718, when he was appointed by Governor Hunter surveyor-general of the colony of New York. He was an eminent naturalist and published in 1720 an account of the climate of the State. In 1735 he wrote a paper on the sore-throat-distemper; and a paper on cancer, published shortly after, is said to have been written by him. Subsequently, in 1743, he published Observations on the Yellow Fever of New York, 1741-'42.[1]

To him is due the credit of suggesting the establishment of the American Philosophical Society. His botanic and other writings exhibit great industry and powers of observation, he having collected and described between three hundred and four hundred new plants. His History of the Five Nations, in two volumes, is the best history of these Indians extant. He held the position of lieutenant-governor in 1761 and again in 1775, besides other positions of honor and trust, and died, September 26, 1776, at the age of 88.

In 1740, Isaac Dubois took the degree of M. D. at Leyden and published a thesis on the "Use and abuse of blood-letting." He practiced in New York, where he died, in 1743.

Dr. John Nicoll died in 1745, after having practiced in the city of New York for nearly half a century. He served as one of the judges of the court in Governor Lesler's time.

John Dupuy was a contemporary of Dr. Nicoll and a man of skill and prominence in the medical profession, but died in 1745, at the early age of 28.

---

[1] American Medical and Philosophical Register, p. 310.

Frank Brinley was a surgeon of the New York provincial troops during the French and Indian war. He went to South Carolina in 1757 or 1758, but died, on his way back, at Shelburne, N. J.

Dr. James Brewer, a native of Massachusetts, practiced at Yorktown during the Revolution. On the night of November 19, 1780, a party of British soldiers surrounded the house of Dr. Ebenezer White, a zealous patriot; but, Dr. White having escaped, they seized upon Dr. Brewer. As the captors and their prisoner were leaving town, they were fired upon, and Dr. Brewer was mortally wounded by his friends, who sought to rescue him, and expired the following day, aged 39 years.

Ebenezer Crosby, a surgeon in the New York Guards of the Continental Army, a native of Quincy, Mass., graduated from Harvard in 1777 and finished his medical education at the University of Pennsylvania. After the war he secured an enviable reputation in New York and in 1785 was elected professor in Columbia College, which appointment he retained until his death, July 16, 1788.

Charles McKnight, of Irish descent, was born at Cranbury, N. J., October 10, 1750; graduated from Princeton in 1771; studied medicine with Dr. Shippen, and entered the Continental Army as a surgeon, but was afterward appointed senior surgeon of the flying-hospital in the middle department. At the close of the war he settled in New York, where he delivered lectures on anatomy and surgery. He communicated a case of extra-uterine abdominal fetus successfully removed by an operation, (see vol. 4, Mem. Med. Society of London.) The doctor was one of the earliest physicians in New York to use a carriage as a conveyance in his rounds to visit patients. He died November 16, 1791, aged 41.

Archibald McDonald, born in Scotland in 1745, came to this country at the age of 12, and resided for some time in Canada. His brother, an officer in the British army, sent him to Philadelphia to acquire a medical education. He commenced practice in North Carolina and subsequently served for several years as a surgeon in the British army. In 1787 he married a lady of Dutchess County and removed to White Plains, where he resided until his death, December 21, 1813. From a genealogical manuscript in the handwriting of his brother, it appears that one of his ancestors married a sister of Robert de Bruce.

Dr. John Thomas, born at Plymouth, Mass., April 1, 1758, entered the Continental Army in 1776, in which he served as surgeon throughout the war. On the termination of hostilities he settled at Poughkeepsie, where he resumed practice with great success. He died in 1818, at the age of 60.

Dr. Ebenezer White, son of Rev. Ebenezer White, was born in Westchester County in 1744 and settled at Yorktown previous to the commencement of the Revolution. He was much interested in politics and religion, possibly at the expense of his progress and proficiency in medicine. During the Revolution he was noted as a patriot, the British making several ineffectual attempts to capture him for the purpose of exchanging him for an English surgeon then in the hands of the Americans. He died, March 8, 1825, at the age of 81.

Dr. Samuel Adams, of Mt. Pleasant, a native of Scotland, came to America about the time of the revolutionary war, and probably served as a surgeon in the Continental Army. After the war he settled in Westchester County. So great was his reputation as a surgeon that for many years no important surgical operation was performed in Westchester or the contiguous counties without his presence. He died in 1828, at the age of 90 years.

Isaac Gilbert Graham, a descendant of the Duke of Montrose, and a son of Dr. Andrew Graham, was born in South Parish, Conn., September 10, 1760; studied medicine under his father, a physician of good standing, and entered the American revolutionay army as an assistant surgeon at an early age. He possessed the warm regard of General Washington and of the officers of the General's staff for his professional ability and staunch patriotism. At the close of the war he married and settled at Unionville, where he practiced for nearly sixty years. Died September 1, 1848, in his eighty-eighth year.

Samuel Osborne, a son of Dr. John Osborne, of Middletown, Conn., studied medicine and became a physician of repute in Brooklyn. He subsequently resided in New York City.

Ebenezer Sage, of Sag Harbor, a graduate of Yale College in 1778, was a practitioner of medicine and a literary and political character of note; also a member of Congress from New York from 1809 to 1815, and died in 1834.

Dr. John Bard, a native of Burlington, N. J., was born February 1, 1716. Having completed his preliminary education, he was apprenticed to Dr. Kearsley, an English surgeon of eminence. After serving his apprenticeship he commenced practice in Philadelphia in 1737, but removed to New York in 1746, at the earnest solicitation of many of the inhabitants of that city, and there practiced until within a year of his death, when he retired to his estate near Poughkeepsie, in 1798. On the organization of the Medical Society of New York, in 1788, he was unanimously chosen president. He died of paralysis, March 30, 1799, in his eighty-third year. He won, and retained, the friendship of Dr. Franklin. He was associated with Dr. Middleton in 1750 in performing the second dissection of a human cadaver recorded in America.

Dr. Jacob Ogden was born at Newark, N. J., in 1721, received the best medical education the colonies afforded, and removed to Jamaica, L. I., where he practiced during the remainder of his life. His death, which took place in his fifty-ninth year, was occasioned by a fall from his horse. He wrote several medical dissertations on the sore-throat-distemper of 1769.

Samuel Bard, M. D., son of Dr. John Bard, was born 1742; died in 1821. He studied medicine with his father, and was then sent to Europe.

His medical degree was received from the University of Edinburgh in 1765. His thesis was " De viribus opii." On his return to the United States he settled to practice in New York, where he soon rose to eminence. In 1769 he proposed resolutions in favor of a public hospital, which led to the erection of the New York Hospital. He was one of the professors of, and assisted in organizing in 1767, the first medical school in the city of New York. He was General Washington's physician and was by contemporary physicians held in high esteem. He published a treatise on croup, and in 1788 a paper on uterine hemorrhage. In 1807 he published a compend of midwifery.

Richard Bayley, M. D., born in 1745, died 1801, was an eminent physician in the city of New York. He was well qualified and of a philosophic turn of mind; studied yellow fever with great care, and published an Essay on Yellow Fever in 1797, with Letters on Yellow Fever in 1798. He published an account of cases of angina trachealis, with mode of cure, in 1781. He is said to have been one of the first physicians who rode to visit their patients.[1]

Dr. Attwood, according to the authority of the historian Watson, was the first physician in New York to devote his time to obstetric practice and to announce himself by advertisement to the public as an obstetrician. He was a contemporary of Dr. Bayley.

Dr. Jacob Ogden, a native of New Jersey, practiced his profession for many years at Jamaica, L. I. He was particularly noted in his day for his advocacy of inoculation and was a successful and intelligent practitioner. He was the author of a number of papers on the malignant sore-throat and other diseases.

Dr. Seth Miller, a native of Pennsylvania, was the first physician to settle in Sing Sing, N. Y.

Nicholas Romayne, M. D., born in the city of New York in 1756, was educated to medicine and rose to eminence. He was elected president in 1807 of the New York State Medical Society. He was a fine scholar and an active promoter of all educational measures. He died July 20, 1817.

Dr. Benjamin Treadwell, a physician of Long Island, was in practice for nearly sixty-five years. He died in North Hampstead in 1830, aged 95.

Dr. Samuel Clossy, a native of Ireland, came to America and settled in New York as early as 1734. He assisted in organizing the medical college in that city and in 1767 was appointed professor of anatomy. He died in Ireland during the revolutionary war.

Peter Middleton, M. D., a native of Scotland, assisted Dr. Bard in his dissection in 1750, the first in the State of New York. He received a professorship in the medical college in 1767. He published a paper on croup and a medical discourse. He died in 1781.

John Jones, M. D., of Welsh extraction, was born at Jamaica, L. I.,

---

[1] Watson's Historic Tales of Olden Times, 1832, p. 123.

in 1729. His father, Evan Jones, was a physician. He studied medicine with Dr. Cadwallader of Philadelphia, but completed his studies in the European schools; settled in New York, and was appointed to the chair of surgery in the Medical College. He served as surgeon in the war of 1755. In 1780 he was in Philadelphia and was the physician to Washington and Franklin. He made many contributions to the department of surgery. He died June 23, 1791, aged 62.

NEW YORK ARMY-SURGEONS IN THE REVOLUTION.

The following medical gentlemen of New York State served as surgeons in the American Army during some portion of the Revolution:

George Campbell, Andrew Cragie, George Draper, John Elliott, Stephen Graham, Henry Moore, Abner Prior, Thomas Reed, Nicholas Schuyler, William P. Smith, Caleb Sweet, Malachi Treat, Samuel Woodruff, and Joseph Young.

Caleb Austin was commissioned, July 1, 1777, in Colonel John Lamb's regiment of New York artillery. John Cochran was director-general of the medical department.

Samuel Cook was commissioned, November 16, 1776, in Colonel Lewis Dubois's regiment, in which he remained till the close of the war.

Elias Cornelius was commissioned in Colonel Israel Angell's regiment of Rhode Island troops, at the age of 19 years, in opposition to the wishes of his parents, who were attached to the British interests in America. He was captured and confined in New York, but made his escape, rejoined the Army, and remained at his post until the latter part of the year 1781. He died, June 13, 1823, at Somers, N. Y., at the age of 65.

Surgeon Mordecai Hale died December 9, 1832.

Ebenezer Hutchinson was commissioned in Colonel Lewis Dubois's regiment, June 12, 1778.

Isaac Ledyard entered the medical department of the Army in March, 1776.

Surgeon Benjamin B. Stockton died June 9, 1829.

Josiah Watrous, commissioned in Colonel Ebenezer Stevens's regiment of artillery September 4, 1777, was stationed at West Point until January 8, 1779, when he resigned.

Surgeon John F. Vacher died December 4, 1807.

William Wheeler, commissioned in 1777, resigned January 8, 1779.

Henlock Woodruff entered the medical department of the Army in 1775

Dr. Peter van der Lynn, a native of Holland, was a surgeon in Colonel Paulding's regiment during the Revolution. In 1777, when Fort Montgomery was attacked, he and General Clinton escaped from being taken prisoners by swimming across the Hudson.

Daniel Menema, a native of New York, served as surgeon in the Second New York Regiment to the close of the war. He was a man of extensive acquirements and of elegant and affable manners. He was a member of the Society of Cincinnati. In 1806 he was president of the Medical Society of Queens County. He died at Jamaica, L. I., January 20, 1810.

Benjamin Welles was surgeon's mate, and then surgeon, from 1777 to the close of the revolutionary war. After the war he settled in Wayne, Steuben County, N. Y., where he practiced with reputation, and died April 19, 1814.

Samuel Stringer, a native of Maryland, having studied medicine, was commissioned in the British army, and was at Quebec in 1758. At the close of the war he settled to practice at Albany, N. Y.

When the revolutionary war commenced, Congress appointed him director-general of hospitals in the northern department. He was a man of ability, but resigned his commission in 1777, and returned to resume a practice which was large and lucrative to the close of his life. He died July 11, 1817, aged 83.

John Thomas, a native of Massachusetts, served as surgeon during the war. After peace was declared he settled and practiced his profession at Poughkeepsie, N. Y., where he died in 1818.

David Shepard, a native of New York, raised and commanded a company at the breaking-out of the Revolution. He resigned the captaincy for the position of surgeon. He was in the battle of Bunker Hill. He died at Amsterdam, Montgomery County, N. Y., December 12, 1818, aged 74.

Nicholas Schuyler, a native of New York, entered the Federal Army as a surgeon at Albany, April 1, 1777. He was an ardent patriot and an active and intelligent surgeon, performing arduous and valuable services during the war. He died at Troy, November 24, 1824.

Thomas Reid was a surgeon of the revolutionary army and during the last two years of the war served in Colonel Luyster's New York regiment. He died at Johnstown, Montgomery County, N. Y., September 18, 1826.

Moses Willard served as surgeon's mate and as surgeon during the war, a portion of the time in Lieutenant-Colonel Willett's regiment.

Moses Younglove was surgeon's mate, and as surgeon served with reputation in various departments. He was a gentleman of varied accomplishments and of fine executive ability, was representative in the legislature, and held other official positions.

Walter Vrooman Whimple was a surgeon in the Revolution. He accompanied the Army to Canada and was actively engaged.

Dr. J. Cochran, of Pennsylvania, studied medicine in Lancaster, Pa., with Dr. Thompson; was a surgeon in the Revolution; after the war settled in Albany; he was on a special reconnaissance, of hardship and danger, of General Washington, April 10, 1777; was appointed surgeon-general of the middle department and in October, 1781, director-general of the hospitals of the United States. He died April 6, 1807, aged 76.

To simply record the names of the many physicians who, prior to the beginning of the present century, rose to eminence in New York, would extend this paper to too great a length. The spirit of legislation[1] in the State has always been liberal and encouraging to the profession.

AFTER THE REVOLUTION.

When the success of the colonies in America became a fact, the serious-minded and provident leaders in public affairs everywhere made liberal provision for education, but rarely further than qualified their sons for becoming ministers and teachers. Colleges were founded and means furnished to a favored few to enable them to attend the universities of England and the Continent. To Oxford, Cambridge, Aberdeen, Leyden, Padua, and Paris, students were sent before the colonies were fifty years old. And, indeed, professional men largely continued to seek their medical education abroad until the beginning of the present century.

Students of divinity often took advantage of their residence in Europe to attend medical lectures and "walk the hospitals," as it was termed; and not a few of them received the doctorate in medicine and afterward became eminently successful in both professions.

---

[1] The following laws were enacted in New York prior to the revolutionary war. The Dutch records show that, February 2, 1652, an order was promulgated regulating the duties of chirurgions. (See Medical Register, City of New York, 1865.)

An act allowing physicians to travel on the Lord's day, enacted 1695, Stat. N. Y., ed. 1691-1751, p. 23; An act exempting physicians and chirurgeons from performing the duties of constable or tax-collector, enacted 1715, Stat. N. Y., ed. 1691-1751, p. 117; Physicians, doctors of physic, practitioners of physic, and surgeons exempt from performing military duty—exempt in case of an invasion—section 23, act 1755, Stat. N. Y., ed. 1752-'63, p. 53; An act to prevent infectious distempers being brought into this colony, and to hinder the spreading thereof, enacted 1755, Stat. N. Y., ed. 1752-'63, p. 157; An act to explain the foregoing act, enacted 1755, Stat. N. Y., ed. 1752-'63, p. 57; An act to continue the same, enacted 1756, Stat. N. Y., ed. 1752-'63, fol. 100; An act to appropriate the money raised by divers lotteries for erecting a college and pest-house, enacted 1756, Stat. N. Y., ed. 1752-'63, p. 111; An act to prevent the bringing in and spreading of infectious distempers in this colony, enacted 1758, Stat. N. Y., ed. 1752-'63, p. 137; An act to regulate the practice of physic and surgery in the city of New York, enacted 1760, Stat. N. Y., ed. 1752-'63, p. 188; An act to revive an act to prevent the bringing in and spreading of infectious distempers in this colony, with an addition thereto regulating the practice of inoculation for the small-pox enacted 1763, Stat. N. Y., ed. 1752-'63, p. 432; An act continuing the foregoing act, enacted 1767, Stat. N. Y., p. 493; An act for the better support of the hospital to be erected in the city of New York for poor and indigent persons, enacted March 24, 1772, Stat. N. Y., ed. 1763-'73, p. 696; An act to prevent infectious distempers in the counties of Westchester, Dutchess, and Orange, and regulating inoculation therein, enacted 1772, Stat. N. Y., ed. 1763-'73, p. 696; An act for regulating the practice of inoculation for the small-pox in the city of Albany, enacted 1773, Stat. N. Y., ed. 1763-'73, p. 720; An act to repeal an act to prevent infectious distempers in the counties of Westchester, Dutchess, and Orange, so far as it relates to the borough and town of Westchester and manor of Phillipsborough, enacted 1773, Stat. N. Y., ed. 1763-'73, p. 791.

HONORS TO MEDICAL MEN.

Dr. John Pott was made temporary head of the government of the colony of Virginia in 1628. Gerardus Beekman, also Cadwallader Colden, both physicians, were acting governors of New York at a later period.

There were five physicians in the Congress that declared the independence of America: Josiah Bartlett, Benjamin Rush, Matthew Thornton, Oliver Wolcott, and Lyman Hall.

The second and third presidents of Harvard and the first of the College of New Jersey were from the ranks of medicine. The numerous high and responsible positions held by professional men before and during the revolutionary war, in Pennsylvania, South Carolina, and other States, show the special fitness of medical men of the period for such trusts.

SMALL NUMBER OF TRAINED PRACTITIONERS.

The duplication of professions and diversity of vocation in the same person served to retard the founding of medical institutions by reducing the number of those possessing special executive talent, who might otherwise have been expected to interest themselves in such enterprises.

The number at any one time of highly educated and pre-eminently skillful physicians in a country has ever been limited and must always be so.

The advantages possessed by these new settlements were not sufficiently attractive to cultured physicians, who had passed through the long courses of training then considered necessary to entitle them to practice the art of healing, to draw them hither in any considerable numbers.

New countries and pioneer settlements are usually overrun by adventurers; indeed, these new fields *invite* the most adventurous and least qualified, to the credit of humanity, and some who were unpleasantly familiar with the processes of the law in their native land became useful and exemplary citizens in the New World.

The public records of that period have frequent allusions to the hordes of charlatans. One writer says: "The quacks abound as the locusts of Egypt." Another says of New York: "That place boasts the honor of above forty gentlemen of the faculty, and far the greatest part of them are mere pretenders to a profession of which they are entirely ignorant."[1]

BEGINNINGS OF LEGISLATIVE PROTECTION.

In Virginia an effort was made to protect the people against excessive charges, and yet encourage educated practitioners. The earliest law enacted in any of the colonies relating to medical men that I have seen

---

[1] New York Independent Reflector, 1753.

is the act passed by the colony of Virginia in 1639. This act was revised in 1645-'46.[1]

In the colony of Connecticut in particular, and in other rural communities, where the empiric seldom repaired, the absurdities of Indian practice became popular.

The earliest fee-bill that I have seen was that established by an act passed by the colony of Virginia, August, 1736, entitled "An act for regulating the fees and accounts for practicers of physic," which allowed a difference of nearly one-half in favor of physicians who had taken a degree in some university over those who had served an apprenticeship only.[2]

---

[1] Whereas by the ninth act of assembly, held the 21st of October, 1639, consideration being had and taken of the immoderate and excessive rates and prices exacted by practitioners in physick and chirurgery, and the complaints made to the then assembly of the bad consequence thereof, it so happening through the said intollerable exactions that the hearts of divers masters were hardened rather to suffer their servants to perish for want of fit means and applications than by seeking relief to fall into the hands of griping and avaricious men; it be apprehended by such masters, who were more swayed by politick respects than Xian (Christian) duty or charity, that it was the more gainfull and saving way to stand to the hazard of their servants than to entertain the certain charge of a physitian or chirurgeon, whose demands for the most parte exceed the purchase of the patient; it was therefore enacted, for the better redress of the like abuses thereafter, untill some fitter course should be advised on, for the regulating physitians and chirurgeons within the colony, that it should be lawful and free for any person or persons in such cases where they should conceive the acco't of the physitian or chirurgeon to be unreasonable, either for his pains or for his druggs or medicines, to arrest the said physitian or chirurgeon either to the quarter-court or county-court where they inhabitt, where the said phisitian should declare upon oath the true value, worth, and quantity of his druggs and medicines administered to or for the use of the plt., (patient,) whereupon the court where the matter was tryed was to adjudge, and allow to the said phisitian or chirurgeon such satisfaction and reward as they in their discretions should think fitt.

And it was further ordered, that when it should be sufficiently proved in any of the said courts that a phisitian or chirurgeon had neglected his patient, or that he had refused, being thereunto required, his helpe or assistance to any person or persons in sickness or extremity, that the said phisitian or chirurgeon should be censured by the said court for such his neglect or refusal, which said act, and every clause therein mentioned and repeated, this present grand assembly to all intents and purposes doth revive, ratifie, allow, and confirme, with this only exception that the plts. (or, patients) shall have their remedy at the county-courts respectively, unless in case of appeal.—Enacted Gr. Assem. Va., sess. 1645-'66, (Hening's Statutes at Large, vol. 1, pp. 316, 317.)

[2] An act for regulating the fees and accounts of the practicers in physic.

I. Whereas the practice of physic in this colony is most commonly taken up and followed by surgeons, apothecaries, or such as have only served apprenticeships to those trades, who often prove very unskilful in the art of a phisician; and yet do demand excessive fees and exact unreasonable prices for their medicines which they administer, and do too often, for the sake of making up long and expensive bills, load their patients with great quantities thereof, than are necessary or useful, concealing all their compositions, as well to prevent the discovery of their practice, as of the true value of what they administer: which is become a grievance, dangerous and intolerable, as well to the poorer sort of people, as others, & doth require the most effectual remedy that the nature of the thing will admit:

Although partial recognition of the profession and protection of the people had been secured in several of the colonies, and particularly in some of the large cities, by legislation, the first well-considered act regulating the practice of physic was that passed in New York, June 10, 1760,[1] which required all practitioners of medicine in the city of New

II. *Be it therefore enacted, by the lieutenant-governor, council, and burgesses of the present general assembly, and it is hereby enacted, by the authority of the same,* That from and after the passing of this act, no practicer in. phisic, in any action or suit whatsoever, hereafter to be commenced in any court of record in this colony, shall recover, for visiting any sick person, more than the rates hereafter mentioned: that is to say—

Surgeons and apothecaries, who have served an apprenticeship to those trades, shall be allowed:

	£	s.	d.
For every visit and prescription in town, or within five miles	0	5	00
For every mile above five and under ten	0	1	00
For every visit of ten miles	0	10	00
And for every mile above ten	0	00	06
With an allowance of all ferriage in their journeys.			
To surgeons, for a simple fracture and cure thereof	2	00	00
For a compound fracture and cure thereof	4	00	60
But those persons who have studied physic in any university, and taken any degree therein, shall be allowed for every visit and prescription in town or within five miles	0	10	00
If above five miles, for every mile more under ten	0	1	00
For a visit, if not above ten miles	1	00	00
And for every mile above ten	0	01	00

With an allowance of ferriages, as before.

III. And to the end the true value of the medicines administered by any practicer in phisic, may be better known, and judged of, *Be it further enacted, by the authority aforesaid,* That whenever any pills, bolus, portion, draught, electuary, decoction, or any medicines, in any form whatsoever, shall be administered to any sick person, the person administering the same shall, at the same time, deliver in his bill, expressing every particular thing made up therein; or if the medicine administered be a simple, or compound, directed in the *dispensatories,* the true name thereof shall be expressed in the same bill, together with the quantities and prices, in both cases. And in failure thereof, such practicer, or any apothecary, making up the prescription of another, shall be nonsuited, in any action or suit hereafter commenced, which shall be grounded upon such bill or bills: Nor shall any book, or account, of any practicer in phisic, or any apothecary, be permitted to be given in evidence, before a court; unless the articles therein contained, be charged according to the direction of this act.

IV. *And be it further enacted, by the authority aforesaid,* That this act shall continue and be in force, for and during two years, next after the passage thereof and from thence to the end of the next session of assembly.—(Hening's Stat. at Large, vol. iv, pp. 509, 510.)

[1] An act to regulate the practice of physick and surgery in the city of New York, passed June 10, 1760.

Whereas many ignorant and unskilful persons in physick and surgery, in order to gain a subsistence, do take upon themselves to administer physick and practice surgery in the city of New York, to the endangering of the lives and limbs of their patients, and many poor and ignorant persons inhabiting the said city, who have been persuaded to become their patients, have been great sufferers thereby; for preventing such abuses for the future—

I. *Be it enacted by his honor the lieutenant-governor, the council, and the general assembly, and it is hereby enacted by the authority of the same,* That from and after the publica-

York to obtain a license certifying qualifications from His Majesty's council, judges of the supreme court, the King's attorney-general, and the mayor of the city.

A general law was passed in New Jersey in 1772,[1] closely patterned

tion of this act no person whatsoever shall practice as a physician or surgeon in the said city of New York before he shall first have been examined in physick and surgery, and approved of and admitted by one of His Majesty's council, the judges of the supreme court, the King's attorney-general, and the mayor of the city of New York for the time being, or by any three or more of them, taking to their assistance for such examinations such proper person or persons as they in their discretion shall think fit. And if any candidate, after due examination of his learning and skill in physick and surgery as aforesaid, shall be approved and admitted to practice as a physician and surgeon, or both, the said examiners, or any three or more of them, shall give, under their hands and seals, to the person so admitted as aforesaid, a testimonial of his examination and admission, and in the form following, to wit:

"To all whom these presents shall come or may concern:

"Know ye, that we, whose names are hereunto subscribed, in pursuance of an act of the lieutenant-governor, and council, and the general assembly, made and published at New York, the tenth day of June, in the year of our Lord one thousand seven hundred and sixty, entitled 'An act to regulate the practice of physick and surgery in the city of New York,' have duly examined ———, physician (or) surgeon, or physician and surgeon, (as the case may be,) and, having approved of his skill, have admitted him as a physician (or) surgeon, (or) physician and surgeon, to practice in the said faculty or faculties throughout this province of New York.

"In testimony whereof we have subscribed our names and affixed our seals to this instrument, at New York, this ——— day of ———, anno Domini one thousand ———."

II. *And be it further enacted by the authority aforesaid*, That if any person shall practice in the city of New York as a physician or surgeon, or both as a physician and surgeon, without such testimonial as aforesaid, he shall, for every such offense, forfeit the sum of five pounds, one-half thereof to the use of the person or persons who shall sue for the same and the other moiety to the church-wardens and vestrymen of the said city for the use of the poor thereof, the said forfeiture to be recovered with costs before the mayor, recorder, or any one of the aldermen of the said city, who are hereby empowered in a summary way to hear, try, and determine any suit brought for such forfeiture, and to give judgment and to award execution thereupon: *Provided*, That this act shall not extend to any person or persons administering physick or practicing surgery within the said city before the publication thereof, or to any person having His Majesty's commission and employed in his service as a physician and surgeon.

[1] An act to regulate the practice of physic and surgery within the colony of New Jersey, passed September 26, 1772.

Whereas many ignorant and unskilful persons in physic and surgery, to gain a subsistence, do take upon themselves to administer physic and practice surgery in the colony of New Jersey, to the endangering of the lives and limbs of their patients, and many of His Majesty's subjects, who have been persuaded to become their patients, have been great sufferers thereby; for the prevention of such abuses for the future:

SECTION I. *Be it enacted by the governor, council, and general assembly, and it is hereby enacted by the same*, That from and after the publication of this act no person whatsoever shall practice as a physician or surgeon within this colony of New Jersey before he shall first have been examined in physic or surgery, approved of and admitted by any two of the judges of the supreme court for the time being, taking to their assistance for such examination such person or persons as they, in their discretion, shall think fit; for which service the said judges of the supreme court, as aforesaid, shall

after that of New York, but more specific and strict in its requirements, placing the licensing power with the supreme court of the State.

be entitled to a fee of twenty shillings, to be paid by the person so applying; and if any candidate, after due examination of his learning and skill in physic and surgery, as aforesaid, shall be approved and admitted to practice as a physician or surgeon, or both, the said examiners, or any two or more, shall give, under their hands and seals, to the person so admitted as aforesaid, a testimonial of his examination and admission in the form following, to wit:

"To all whom these presents shall come or may concern:

"Know ye, that we whose names are hereunto subscribed, in pursuance of an act of the governor, council, and general assembly of the colony of New Jersey, made in the twelfth year of the reign of our sovereign lord King George the Third, entitled 'An act to regulate the practice of physic and surgery within the colony of New Jersey,' having duly examined ———, of ———, physician or surgeon, or physician and surgeon, to practice in the said faculty or faculties throughout the colony of New Jersey. In testimony whereof we have hereunto subscribed our names, and affixed our seals to this instrument, at ———, this day of ———, annoque Domini 17—."

SEC. 2. *And be it further enacted by the authority aforesaid*, That if any person or persons shall practice as a physician or surgeon, or both, within the colony of New Jersey without such testimonial as aforesaid, he shall forfeit and pay for every such offence the sum of five pounds; one-half thereof to the use of any person or persons who shall sue for the same, and the other half to the use of the poor of any city or township where such persons shall so practice contrary to the tenor of this act, to be recovered in any court where sums of this amount are cognizable, with costs of suit.

SEC. 3. * * * *Provided always*, That this act shall not be construed to extend to any person or persons administering physic or practicing surgery before the publication hereof, within this colony, or to any person bearing His Majesty's commission and employed in his service as a physician and surgeon: *And provided always*, That nothing in this act shall be construed to extend to hinder any person or persons from bleeding, drawing teeth, or giving assistance to any person, for which services such persons shall not be entitled to make any charge or receive any reward: *Provided also*, That nothing herein contained be construed to hinder any skilful physician or surgeon from any of the neighboring colonies being sent for, upon any particular occasion, from practicing on such occasions within this colony.

SEC. 4. *And be it further enacted by the authority aforesaid*, That any person now practicing physic or surgery, or that shall hereafter be licensed as by this act is directed, shall deliver his account or bill of particulars to all and every patient in plain English words, or so nearly so as the articles will admit of; all and every of which accounts shall be liable, whenever the patient, his executors, or administrators shall require, to be taxed by any one or more of the judges of the inferior court of common pleas of the county, city, or borough wherein the party complaining resides, calling to their assistance such persons therein skilled as they may think proper.

SEC. 5. *And be it further enacted by the authority aforesaid*, That every physician, surgeon, or mountebank doctor who shall come into and travel through this colony, and erect any stage or stages for the sale of drugs or medicines of any kind, shall for every such offence forfeit and pay the sum of twenty pounds, proclamation-money, to be recovered in any court where the same may be cognizable, with costs of suit; one-half to the person who will prosecute the same to effect, the other half to the use of the poor of any city, borough, township, or precinct where the same offence shall be committed.

SEC. 6. *And be it further enacted by the authority aforesaid*, That this act, and every clause and article herein contained, shall continue and be in force for the space of five years, and from thence until the end of next session of the general assembly, and no longer.—(Laws of New Jersey, folio-edition, 1776, p. 376.)

RISE OF HOSPITALS.

Hospitals,[1] or institutions similar in character to the infirmaries of the

[1] The word "hospital" is derived from the latin *hospes*, a guest, a stranger. "Hostel" and "hotel" have the same derivation. A hospital in cloisters was an extra apartment or room, a place of shelter for strangers, equivalent in purpose to our hotel, to the ξενοδοχεῖ of the Greeks and the *hospitium* of the Romans. Although it is to the Christians that we must look for the full development of institutions having for their purpose the care of the poor and the sick, still the germs of all our benevolent institutions seem to have had an existence among the ancient Egyptians, Greeks, and Romans. The sick were treated in the first temple erected to Esculapius as early as 1134 B. C., at Titanus, a city of Peloponnesus. Young candidates for the priestly office were also taught in them the practice of medicine. The temple of Esculapius, at Cos, being the most famous, had accommodations for the sick. It is probable that the institution established by Antoninus at Epidorus, a hundred years before Christ, was of the same character. One existed on the island of the Tiber at Rome, to which sick slaves were taken to be healed. There was a public building at Delos, on the island Rhenæa, of the character of a hospital, which was occupied by aged women. At a later period, buildings seem to have been erected near the temples for the accommodation of sick persons visiting them. At Jerusalem there was a large building named Bethesda, or "a house of mercy," for the accommodation of the infirm.

The term "hospital" is first used in connection with curative establishments in the works of St. Jerome.

The first hospital which attained any permanent celebrity was established and richly endowed by the Emperor Valens, at Cæsarea, between the years 370 and 380 A. D.

To either St. Ephraim, who died in 381, or St. Fabiola, is due the credit of founding infirmaries, which were supported by charitable contributions, for the exclusive purpose of treating the sick. The good Bishop Nonus, at Edessa, in Mesopotamia, founded a hospital in 460. Another was opened at Rome about the same time.

The *Taberna Meritoria*, at Rome, seems to have been occupied as a sort of asylum for invalids. Hospitals for the poor and the sick were much encouraged by the early Christians. The council of Nice, A. D. 325, speaks of them as institutions well known, and deserving support and encouragement. St. Chrysostom established a hospital at Constantinople towards the close of the fourth century. Basilius established a hospital in Cappadocia in 370. Paula, a rich Christian lady of Rome, established one about the same year in Jerusalem. In Rome alone, in the ninth century, there were twenty-four hospitals. Alexius Comnenus, in the eleventh century, established hospitals for invalid soldiers at Constantinople. The Hôtel des Invalides of Paris and the Chelsea Hospital of England are of this character. The Hôtel-Dieu in Paris was founded about the middle of the seventh century; Hospitaliers de Saint Antoine de Viennois, in 1198; l'Hôpital des Petites Maisons, 1564; the Hôpital de la Charité, 1602; Hôpital St. Louis, 1607; Notre Dame de la Pitié, 1612; Hospice de l'Accouchement, 1625; Hospice Incurables Femmes, 1634; Hospice Bicolri, 1634, as a retreat for disabled soldiers; La Maison de Charian, 1641; Hospice des Enfants Trouvés, 1656; Hospice de la Salpêtrière, 1656. In Germany, the Hospital of the Holy Ghost and St. George's Hospital, in Bern, were established as early as 1208; St. Gertrude Hospital, 1405, remodeled in 1734; Hospes pour les Enfans, 1687; Hôtel de Refuge, 1699; Maison d'Orange, 1704; Charité, 1710; Invalid House, 1748.

From allusions in history, it is almost certain that institutions known as hospitals were maintained at other important localities for the accommodation of travelers or the sick requiring attention. A foundling-hospital was established at Milan in 787, and a hospital for orphans at Constantinople in 1090. The earliest hospital founded in Great Britain was St. Bartholomew's, in 1122; but, for the three centuries that followed, no other of note was founded in that empire. In the sixteenth century, two institutions were ounded in Great Britain: one, Bethlehem, commonly called Bedlam, (1547,) for lunatics,

present time, have probably existed from an early period in the world's history, and certainly from about the period that Christian charity was taught by its divine Master in person.

It was not, however, until the eleventh or twelfth century that hospitals specially intended for the care of the sick became popular and recognized institutions important to large cities.

During the Middle Ages every monastery had its almonry, where onetenth of its revenues were dispensed to the poor and sick; hence the origin in many instances of the almshouse, from which grew up the infirmary and pharmacy. The monks were our earliest botanists, and in their gardens grew not only table-vegetables, but medicinal plants; and in distribution of these for the benefit of the sick may be traced the earliest development of the office of the dispensary and the apothecary of the present day.[1]

---

and St. Thomas's, (1553,) as a general hospital. There were none established in Great Britain in the seventeenth century. In the eighteenth century, however, there were twelve founded by that nation, and an act of Parliament in 1729 levied a tax of sixpence on each seaman trading in America, for the support of the Royal Hospital.[*]

Twenty-three have been founded during the first half of the present century. From the slow rise of hospitals proper in Europe, it will not seem strange that they developed into a system but slowly in America. In 1639 there was a small hospital established at Quebec, which was probably the earliest in America. In 1658 one existed in New Amsterdam. In 1701, the year the first settlement was made at Detroit, a "pest-house" was provided for at Salem, Mass., and in 1717 a hospital for contagious diseases was built at Boston, in the same State. In 1751 the Pennsylvania Hospital, at Philadelphia, was chartered, with a department for the care of the insane. The hospital of the city of New York was chartered in 1771. In 1772 the Eastern Lunatic Hospital, at Williamsburg, Va., was chartered. Since then they have multiplied so steadily that, besides extensive State-hospitals for the insane, there are found, in every large city of the Union and in almost all of our chief towns, institutions of this class for the treatment of disease, for the relief of infirmities, and for the proper care of wounds. It is to such curative establishments that the term "hospital" is usually restricted in this country, though in Great Britain, as in Europe generally, it is applied indiscriminately to nearly all charitable institutions.

[1] The term "apothecary" is derived from the Greek ἀποθήκη, shop or store. The keeper of a warehouse, or magazine, was formerly called an apothecary. During the early periods of history, physicians undoubtedly prepared their own medicines; but, in the progress of time, and the development of the sciences in every country, it seems to become necessary, or at least adds to the convenience of the physician, to intrust the preparation of medicine to the hands of persons skilled as apothecaries or pharmacists Galen had, in Rome, a drug-shop in the Via Sacra, which was destroyed by fire in the reign of Commodus, about A. D. 181, when the Temple of Peace and other edifices were destroyed. The art of preparing medicines became a distinct branch in Alexandria, in Egypt, towards the beginning of the fourth century B. C., and to it some physicians devoted themselves. It continued as the employment of particular individuals, and thus the pursuit of the physician became separated from the art of the apothecary. Mantias, a pupil of Herophilus in Alexandria, is credited with being the author of the first pharmacopœia. Heras, of Cappadocia, wrote a work on pharmacy, (B. C. 49.) Throughout the East, but particularly in Alexandria, where learning of various kinds was cultivated to a high degree, the study of chemistry and pharmacy was principally

[*] Penn's Archives, vol. i., p. 251.

There is no better index to the actual condition of civilization and the development of Christian charity among a people in any age than the care they take of their sick and destitute. One of the complaints of the settlers in New Amsterdam to the home-government, in 1649, was that they had no hospitals or asylums for the poor, the aged, and sick.[1]

These complaints must have been effective, for an institution, serving this purpose, and known as the Old Hospital or the Five Houses, was sold by the governor of New York in 1680 for £200, after it had become unserviceable and better buildings had been supplied.

---

pursued by the Arabians. The caliph Almansor (754 A. D.) is said to have founded in Bagdad the first public apothecary or drug-shop.

In the thirteenth and fourteenth centuries persons who prepared preserves and confectionery at court or for the nobility, according to formulas, were known by this name. Apothecaries, as compounders of medicines, were first legally established in Italy by an edict of Frederick II, for the Kingdom of Naples, about 1220. Edward III, in 1345, conferred a pension of sixpence a day upon Coursus de Gangeland, an apothecary of London, in recognition of his attendance upon him during an illness in Scotland. This is the first notice of the recognition of an apothecary in England. In 1457 a patent was granted for establishing an apothecary in Stuttgart. In France the statute authorizing the apothecaries was issued in August, 1484, by Charles VIII. Until 1511 no distinctive law was made in Great Britain to distinguish between the different branches of the profession of medicine. In 1540 four physicians were appointed to examine all "wares, drugs, and stuffs" sold by apothecaries. The apothecaries were incorporated by James I, April 9, 1606, being united with 'grocers, from whom they were separated by a new act in 1617. Up to 1815 their authority was confined to London, after which it was extended to England and Wales. This corporation has the power to confer licenses on its members, who are thus invested with the right to administer medicine as well as to prepare and sell it in the shops. Thus a large portion of the practitioners of Great Britain are only apothecaries. The Royal College of Surgeons in London has also a charter and the right to grant diplomas, which are, however, honorary and confer no right to practice. In France the old corporation of apothecary-druggists has dissolved, and a corporation of *pharmaciens* has taken its place, but simply as compounders of medicines. This is true, also, of Italy, Prussia, and Germany. In our own country there is no law defining or limiting the sphere of the vocation of the apothecary.

The United States Pharmacopœia came into existence in the following manner:

In 1816 Lyman Spalding, M. D., of Cornish, N. H., conceived the idea of compiling a national pharmacopœia for use in the United States, and in January, 1817, submitted his project to the New York City Medical Society, with a view to secure the co-operation and authority of all medical societies and colleges for the perfection of the work. He suggested that a convention in each of the four grand geographical divisions of our country be held, and that each adopt a pharmacopœia, which should be submitted to a convention, to meet in the city of Washington, to revise and complete the work. The convention assembled and perfected in a most acceptable manner their laborious work. A regulation was at the same time adopted that a convention should meet in that city every ten years for the revision of the National Pharmacopœia, which was adopted and has been pursued ever since. The National Pharmacopœia, better known as the Pharmacopœia of the United States of America, has, since 1833, been known chiefly as "Wood & Bache's United States Dispensatory." These authors state that they have adopted as a basis for their work the general arrangement agreed upon by the national convention in the pharmacopœia. Decennially a general revision of it is made, which incorporates all the new therapeutic agents of importance, thus keeping it even with the times.

[1] New York Colonial Records.

This was probably the first hospital within the boundaries of the United States. The first general hospital chartered in the colonies was the Pennsylvania Hospital at Philadelphia, in 1751. There was a provision in the charter for the care of the insane, which has since been extended to two large State-institutions for this class. In 1769 measures were taken in New York for the establishment of a general hospital, which was chartered in June, 1771.

Dr. Samuel Bard deserves the honor of suggesting this public charity. The Eastern Lunatic Asylum at Williamsburgh, Va., chartered in 1772 and opened the following year, was the first special and independent institution in this country for the care of the insane. This completes the list of chartered hospitals under colonial rule, although post and temporary military hospitals had previously existed for the treatment of soldiers and other employés of the government in the several colonies.

Provisions of a temporary character, for the treatment of contagious diseases, and especially of small-pox, were made from time to time, as emergencies demanded, by all the colonies; and in some provisions were made for the establishment of permanent inoculating-hospitals.

A pest-house, on Sullivan's Island, near Charleston, S. C., was swept off by a flood in 1752, with fifteen persons in it, some of whom were drowned.[1]

The Philadelphia Dispensary, for the distribution of medicines among the poor, was opened in 1786 and that of New York chartered in 1791.

AUTOPSY.

Dissections were seldom performed prior to 1760, except by stealth, and even an autopsy was rarely permitted, except when suspicion had arisen that death was the result of foul play. In 1690 Governor Slaughter, of New York, died suddenly, and a post-mortem examination was made by Dr. Johannes Kerfbyle, assisted by five other physicians, to determine if he had been poisoned, which is the first recorded case. The detailed statement of the physicians employed in this autopsy gives evidence that they possessed a good degree of proficiency for such investigations.[2]

---

[1] Ramsay's History of South Carolina.

[2] The taking of the testimony of medical men as experts by coroners' juries and criminal courts, in cases of sudden or violent death, is of much more recent practice than might be inferred. The first criminal code in Europe that contained statutory provisions directing the taking of medical testimony in all cases where death was occasioned by violent means was formed or adopted by Charles the Fifth, at Ratisbonne, in 1532. This code laid the foundation for legalized autopsies in criminal cases, for it is only by such means that the medical man, who is sworn by the coroner "diligently to inquire how and in what manner the deceased came to his death," can answer knowingly and correctly.

The office of coroner is first mentioned in a charter granted in the year 925 A. D. by King Athelston to the authorities of Beverly. The powers and duties of coroners are defined and provided for in the common law and in special enactments of the different States.

MIDWIFERY.

Up to about the middle of the eighteenth century the practice of midwifery, as it was called, was exclusively in the hands of women, medical men being called in only in difficult and protracted cases.

Dr. John Maubray is considered to have been the first public teacher of midwifery in Great Britain. His first work was published in 1723.

Dr. James Lloyd, who settled in Boston in 1754, was the first regularly-educated physician in Massachusetts to devote himself to obstetrical practice.

Dr. Attwood is said to have been the first physician in New York to publicly announce himself as devoting himself to the practice of obstetrics. This was in 1762, some years anterior to the revolutionary war

Dr. William Shippen, jr., immediately on his return from the leading European schools, devoted much of his time and ability to this branch of the profession, in Philadelphia, and was the first public teacher of midwifery in America.

In South Carolina this department of practice was first assumed by Dr. John Moultrie, who commenced practice in Charleston as early as 1733, and for forty years was the most celebrated physician and popular obstetrician in the State or in the South. It is probable that his devotion to obstetrics antedates that of any other physician in America.

THE PHYSICIAN AND THE APOTHECARY.

Dr. John Morgan, of Philadelphia, was in 1765 the first American physician to adopt and publicly advocate the theory that medical men should confine themselves to prescribing remedies, leaving to the apothecary the compounding of medicines. This system was gradually adopted in the cities and large towns, and remains the general practice of the regular profession, except in the remoter country-districts.

This division of labor only became an established practice in Great Britain about 1750. In 1754 the College of Physicians and Surgeons passed an act prohibiting their fellows and licentiates taking upon themselves the duties of the apothecary and in 1765 issued an order against the pursuit of specialties.

Even in the larger towns during colonial times medical practice was laborious and unremunerative. The physician often had to ride from 20 to 100 miles on horseback to see a patient. It was at a comparatively late date that the doctor's gig or "chair" was introduced, even into cities. The compounding of prescriptions and the selling of drugs was then often necessary to the country-doctor, and to some extent is still so, but has been pretty generally eliminated from the other duties of the physician in the towns.

FEES.

In rural regions the physician's fees were often paid, if paid at all, in farm-produce, and his remuneration was so uncertain that he was frequently obliged to combine farming with his professional vocation. This was also true of the clerical profession at that period, as farm- or glebe-lands was attached to nearly all the colonial churches.

In fact, in those earlier days of the Republic, a single industrial pursuit could seldom be relied upon for a livelihood, and success and thrift were frequently proportionate to the diversity of occupation; whatever the principal one might be, the second was ordinarily agriculture. The instances were few where medical men in the United States prior to the Revolution acquired large fortunes solely from their professional vocation. It is true that we had many wealthy physicians, but their fortunes were generally acquired by inheritance or by judicious investments and fortunate speculations.

MEDICAL TITLES.[1]

The title of the medical practitioner is not the same in all countries, and the popular meaning of words and titles has so changed that the original signification is, in some instances, almost lost. Thus, in English history we have record of the following appellations having been used: Physician, leech, mire or myre, barbers, barber-surgeon, chirurgeon, surgeon, and doctor. Neither surgeons nor physicians of the present

---

[1] The appellations or terms by which physicians have been known at different periods in different countries are sufficiently curious to merit comment. The words "doctor" and "physician," though of classical origin and occurring in all the languages of Western Europe in a more or less modified form, have in the English language alone acquired their peculiar application to the practitioners and professors of the healing art.

The term "physician" is of Greek origin, being derived from $\varphi\acute{v}\sigma\iota\varsigma$, nature. From the Greek it was transplanted into the Latin and thence into the Italian, Spanish, Portuguese, Provençal, French, German, and English. But both in the original Greek and all the derivative languages, except the English, the word has retained its proper signification, that of "naturalist," "natural philosopher," or "chemist." The word "physician" in French is never used in the sense in which we exclusively use the corresponding English term. And, singularly enough, the word "physician" in English has entirely lost its original meaning and appertains wholly to the medical fraternity. The fact that in the middle ages the functions of the medical practitioner were united with those of the priest, the chemist, and the apothecary, and that the professor of the healing art was almost the only one conversant with the operations of physical nature to the extent of the knowledge of those days, was probably the cause and occasion whence arose the peculiar application of the term in our language.

The word "doctor" has shared almost the same fate. It is a Latin word, derived from *doceo*, to teach; and, both in its parent tongue and through all its derivations in the so-called Latin or Romanic languages, it has retained its original and appropriate meaning, that of *teacher*. To the English tongue alone is confined the use of the term as applicable to the medical practitioner; and with us it has become the most common designation for that purpose, though it has not lost its original meaning entirely or as exclusively as has the word "physician."

The Hebrew word for *physician* was רֹפֵא, (*rōphē*,) from the verb meaning *to sew, to mend*. Gesenius, in giving examples of the application of the word, records Luther's joke, in which he calls physicians "*unseres Herrn Gottes Schuster*"—the cobblers of the

day in Great Britain are called doctors, but are spoken of as surgeon or Mr.* In the United States, however, they are almost invariably denominated doctor.

The earliest date at which we find the title Dr. substituted for surgeon and physician in America is in New England, about 1769. Since that period it has become common throughout the United States, and the popular appellation of "doctor" is now almost exclusively given by Lord God. The Greek ἰατρος is from ιαω, to heal; the Latin *medicus*, from *medeor*, also meaning to heal or to cure; and from the Latin come immediately the Spanish and Italian *medico* and the French *médecin*.

In the twelfth century, in France, according to Collette, practitioners of medicine were commonly called "myres," an appellation which continued to be used for several centuries. It was also in popular use in England. Its derivation has been traced both to the Greek and the Latin languages: Latin, *mirus*, admirable, extraordinary; and Greek, μύρον, an ointment.

Our earliest English or Anglo-Saxon appellation for the physician (also often applied to the priestly office) was the word "leech," from the Saxon *laec*, one who provides, who cures, and the active verb *lacenian*, to treat with medicaments, to heal.

"Her words prevailed, and then the learned *leech*,
His cunning hand 'gan to his wounds to lay,
And all things else the which his art did teach."
—*Spenser, Faerie Queene.*

"The hoary, wrinkled *leech* has watched and toiled,
Tried every health-restoring herb and gum,
And wearied out his painful skill in vain."
—*Rowe.*

This term appears to have been the one in common use, not only during the Anglo-Saxon period of English history, but for a considerable time after the Norman invasion. It is yet common enough in poetry, but not often found out of it in that acceptation. Its disuse was due to the same cause which occasioned the supersedure of many other Anglo-Saxon words: the introduction of Norman, French, and Latin appellations. The medical practitioner then began to be styled "physician" among the educated classes and "doctor" by those in the lower ranks of society, a distinction which yet obtains to a considerable extent.

The English language is full of instances of words which have lost their proper significance and have been appropriated to uses beyond the scope of their original meaning. There is, perhaps, no more remarkable instance of this deflection than the title of doctor; and it is curious to trace the cause of it.

Both the words "physician" and "doctor" are of frequent use in Shakespeare, and to the same purpose as at the present time. King James's Bible, published in 1582, which is followed in this respect by the Catholic version known as the Douay, and all subsequent versions, never uses the word "doctor" in the sense of a medical practitioner. It is not found at all in the translation of the Old Testament; but in that of the New Testament it occurs several times; never in the meaning of a professor of the healing art, but uniformly and invariably in its more natural meaning of *teacher;* that is, *teacher of the law,* (of Moses,) a title somewhat analogous to our title of doctor of divinity.

The word "physician" occurs both in the Old and New Testaments in the same sense which we attribute to it now. The most ancient allusion to members of the medical faculty, and perhaps the earliest mention of them in any historical record extant occurs in Genesis, chap. 50, verse 2, where it is stated that Joseph employed them to embalm the body of his father, preparatory to its transmission to the ancestral burying-place of his family, near the ancient city of Hebron.

the people to the medical practitioner, when speaking *to* him, and the term physician used more generally when speaking *of* him.

MEDICINE IN THE SOUTH.

The Carolinas, from a comparatively early period, furnished numerous valuable contributions to the literature of medicine and natural history, and for some years led all the States in the study of the natural sciences.

As early as 1738, Doctors Maubray, surgeon in the British navy, and Kirkpatrick introduced and conducted successfully general inoculation at Charleston. The practice was at various times resorted to subsequently.

John Lining, a native of Scotland, who settled in Charleston in 1730, was an accomplished physician, and published in 1743 Observations on the Weather of Charleston and, later, An Account of the Excretions of the Human Body. In 1753 he published, in the second volume of the Medical Observations and Inquiries, p. 370, "A description of the American yellow fever." He died in 1760, aged 52 years.

Dr. William Bull was the first native South Carolina physician of note, and the first American, who received the degree of M. D. This was granted at Leyden in 1734, his thesis being on "Colica pictonum." He died July 4, 1791, aged 82.

Lionel Chalmers, a native of Scotland and a well-educated physician, settled in Charleston prior to 1740. In 1754 he published An Essay on Opisthotonos and Tetanus and in 1768 an article on fevers, in which he adopted the "spasmodic theory." In 1776 he published a work in two volumes on the Weather and Diseases of South Carolina. He died in the year 1777, at the age of 62.

Dr. John Moultrie was the next South Carolinian who received the degree of M. D., which was granted in 1749, from Edinburgh. His thesis was "De febra flava."

For the ten years intervening between 1768 and 1778, there were ten natives of South Carolina who received the degree of doctor of medicine at Edinburgh. Various unsuccessful attempts had been made to regulate the practice of medicine in the State.

Alexander Gardner, a native of Edinburgh, settled in Charleston in 1750. In 1754 he wrote a description of a new plant, *Gardenia*, which is published in the first volume of Medical Observations and Enquiries, p. 1. In 1764 he published an account of the *Spigelia mary landica*, or Carolina pink-root, and in 1772 a second and enlarged edition of the paper in the philosophical transactions. He died in London in 1792, aged 64.

Vaccination was introduced into South Carolina in February, 1802, by Dr. David Ramsey, who was one of the most eminent physicians of his day and was several times elected to the State- and national legisatures. During the absence of President Hancock, at which time Dr.

Ramsey occupied a seat in Congress, he was appointed president *pro tempore* of that body, and filled the chair until the return of Mr. Hancock—nearly a year. He was born in Pennsylvania in 1749, graduated at Princeton in 1765, and in 1772 received the degree of M. B. at Philadelphia. He wrote a number of historical works of decided merit and also served as a surgeon in the Continental Army.[1] He died from the effects of a pistol-shot, fired by one Anson More, in May, 1815.

CAROLINA SURGEONS IN THE REVOLUTION.

The following physicians of South Carolina served in a professional capacity in the Continental Army:

Samuel J. Axon, Robert Brownfield, Nathan Brownson, John Carne, Peter Fayssoux, Henry C. Flagg, Oliver Hart, James Houston, Charles Lockman, James Martin, William Neufville, Joseph Prescott, Jesse H. Ramsey, William Read, Sylvester Springer, William S. Stevens, Frederick Gunn, Benjamin Tetard, Thomas T. Tucker, Samuel Vickers, and John Wallace.

David Oliphant served a short time as deputy director-general of the Army, but it is probable that he resigned in 1776, as he was appointed to a judgeship in that year. He was afterward elected to the State assembly of South Carolina.

---

[1] A Review of the Improvements and Progress of Medicine in the Eighteenth Century.

In the Carolinas the following enactments were made by the colonial governments: An act relating unto the office and duty of a coroner, and settling and ascertaining the fees of same, enacted 1706, Stat. S. C., vol. 2, p. 269; An act for the more effectual preventing the spreading of contagious distempers, enacted 1712, Stat. S. C., vol. 2, p. 383; An act for preventing as much as may be the spreading of contagious distempers, enacted 1721, Stat. S. C., vol. 3, p. 127; An act for the better preventing the spreading of the infection of small-pox in Charleston, enacted 1738, Stat. S. C., vol. 3, p. 513; Acts additive to the act for preventing as much as may be the spreading of contagious distempers, enacted 1747, 1752, Stat. S. C., vol. 3, pp. 694-771; An act to prevent the spreading of infectious and contagious distempers in Charleston enacted 1749, Stat. S. C., vol. 3, p. 720; An act for the further preventing the spreading of contagious and malignant distempers in this province, enacted 1752, Stat. S. C., vol. 3, p. 773; An act appropriating for a pest-house and other purposes, enacted 1754, Stat. S. C., vol. 4, p. 10; An act for preventing as much as may be the spreading of contagious and malignant distempers in this province, and repealing the former acts heretofore made for that purpose, enacted 1759, Stat. S. C., vol. 4, p. 78; An act for preventing as much as may be the continuance of the small-pox in, Charleston, and the further spreading of that distemper in this province, enacted 1760, Stat. S. C., vol. 4, p. 106; An act for preventing as much as may be the spreading of the small-pox, enacted 1764, Stat. S. C., vol. 4, p. 182; An act reviving and amending the act of 1759, Stat. S. C., vol. 4, p. 572; An act appointing coroners, enacted 1715, Stat. N. C., ed. 1791, p. 10; An act to prevent malignant and infectious distempers being spread by shipping, importing distempered persons into this province, and other purposes, enacted 1755, Stat. N. C., ed. 1791, p. 170; An act to oblige vessels having contagious distempers on board to perform their quarantine enacted 1774, Stat. N. C., ed. 1791, p. 270; Statute de officio coronatoris, English statute in force in North Carolina, p. 13; Statute for the relief and ordering of persons infected with the plague, English statute in force in North Carolina, p. 353.

Robert Rose and Surgeon Vaughn served to the close of the war, in a regiment formed by the consolidation of the first and second regiments of South Carolina troops.

Dr. Louis Mattel, a native of France and a well-educated physician, practiced near Monks Corner, in South Carolina, for many years. In 1756 he removed to Charleston and practiced in partnership with Dr. Savage. He died about the year 1775.

Joseph Rush, a native of Pennsylvania, a physician of the Revolution, settled after the war to practice on St. John's Island, S. C. He served as surgeon under Commodore Barry. His death took place December 20, 1817.

Alexander Baron, a native of Scotland, a graduate of Edinburgh, in 1768, immigrated to America and settled in Charleston the following year. His acquirements attracted attention, and Drs. Millengen, Oliphant, and Wilson, practitioners of extensive business at the time, assisted to introduce him. He died in Charleston, July 9, 1819, aged 74.

John Lochman, a surgeon of the Revolution, died in Charleston, August 16, 1819. He was a member of the Society of Cincinnati.

Dr. William Butler, a native of South Carolina, was a physician of distinction in the Edgefield district. He was the father of Hon. A. P. Butler. He died November 15, 1821, aged 67.

Tucker Harris, M. D., a native of Charleston, S. C., studied medcine with Lionel Chalmers, in Charleston. He received his medical de gree at Edinburgh. On the breaking-out of the war he entered the mil tary service as a surgeon, and continued in this position until the restoration of peace. He died July 6, 1821, aged 76.

Robert Wilson and his son Samuel were practitioners of reputation during two generations in Charleston. The latter died April, 1827, aged about 70.

William Read, a surgeon in the Revolution, died at Charleston April 20, 1845, aged 91. He was appointed by Congress, May 15, 1781, hospital-physician for the department of the South.

Lyman Hall, a native of Connecticut, a graduate of Yale College of 1747, having studied medicine, settled in Burke County, Ga. He afterward became governor of the State. He was an ardent patriot during the Revolution, and was sent by St. John's parish to the Continental Congress in 1775 and had the honor of signing the immortal document that signalized our independence.

NORTH CAROLINA.

The materials for a medical history of this State are few. Neither the population, the character of her public institutions, the size of her cities, nor the operations of the revolutionary war centered much within her boundaries.

Hugh Williamson, M. D., a native of Pennsylvania, a man of extensive information and fine professional acquirements, was an ardent and influential patriot in the Revolution; was a surgeon in the militia under General Caswell; was a member of Congress and also a member of the convention that framed the Constitution of the United States. He displayed his abilities as an able writer upon every subject that he handled. He died in the city of New York in 1819, aged 83.

James Brehm, during the revolutionary war a surgeon in the infant navy, was a skillful physician of a philosophic turn of mind and a taste for scientific studies. He practiced his profession with success for nearly forty years at Warrenton, where he died, April 8, 1819, at an advanced age.

Lancelot Johnson, a surgeon of the Revolution, died in Caswell County, N. C., September 19, 1832. He served in the Ninth North Carolina Regiment, which was employed chiefly in the South.

Robert Williams died in Pitt County, N. C., October 12, 1840, aged 82. He had served as a surgeon in the Revolution. He was an able physician and a gentleman of superior intelligence and ability. His public services were numerous, and he took part in the committee from North Carolina that ratified the Constitution of the United States.

Nathaniel Alexander, of North Carolina, graduated from Princeton in 1776, and, having studied medicine, entered the Army as a surgeon's mate. Upon the termination of the war he settled at the High Hills of the Santee, where he practiced. He subsequently removed to Mecklenburg, was elected to Congress, and while occupying a seat in that body was chosen governor by the legislature of his State. He died at Salisbury, March 8, 1808, in the fifty-second year of his age.

The following medical men of North Carolina rendered assistance to the American revolutionary army in their professional capacity:

Joseph Blyth, James Fergus, James W. Green, and Solomon Holling.

Surgeon Samuel Curtis died March 31, 1822, in Hillsboro' County.

David Love was surgeon of the North Carolina brigade and was captured by the enemy August 1, 1781, and confined in New York.

William McClure and William McLain entered the Army as early as 1775 or 1776. He died at Lincoln, N. C., October 25, 1828.

EARLY MEDICAL TRAINING IN NEW ENGLAND.

Though the New England States did not lead in medical education their chronicles contain the earliest authentic mention of medical matters and instruction in America.

Giles Firmin, as early as 1647, it would seem, delivered lectures or readings on human osteology, and is said to have had the first "anatomy" in the country, "which he did make and read upon very well." Dr. Firmin returned to England in 1654, was ordained a minister, and died in 1697, aged 80 years.[1]

In 1771, twelve years before the medical department was organized, a

---

[1] New England Historical and Geneological Registers, vol. iv, p. 11.

number of undergraduates of Harvard banded themselves together for the secret study of practical anatomy. Secrecy was a necessity, as dissection and desecration were, in those days, synonymous in the minds of the people. In Massachusetts, and perhaps other States, the practice was a felony for sixty years later.

Who the instructor of this class was is left to conjecture. Possibly it was Joseph Warren, afterward the hero of Bunker Hill. He had recently completed his medical apprenticeship of seven years, according to the usage of the period, and was beginning to practice in Boston. His brother John, in 1783, was instrumental in founding the medical department of Harvard University and was also a member of the senior-class referred to.

CONNECTICUT PHYSICIANS.

Phineas Fiske, born at Milford, Conn., practiced medicine at Haddam, Conn., where he died, 1738, aged 85. He was the fourth graduate of Yale College in 1704. He was a minister and contemporary with Dr. Jared Eliot and distinguished for his skill and success in curing epilepsy and insanity.

Moses Bartlett practiced medicine in Portland, Conn., for over 30 years and died in 1766. He was the son-in-law of Dr. Phineas Fiske, with whom he studied both medicine and theology.

Abijah Moores practiced medicine for many years at Haddam, Conn., where he died in 1759.

Eliot Rawson, a native of Dorchester, Mass., practiced medicine with success for many years at Haddam, Conn., where he died in 1770.

Thomas Levenworth, a native of Connecticut, died at Woodbury, where he practiced for years. He died in 1673.

James Hurlburt, a native of Berlin, Conn., died at Wethersfield, April 11, 1774, aged 56. He was a man of genius and learning, but towards the close of his life became addicted to the extreme use of opium. He was a favorite preceptor for some years with young men studying medicine, all of whom retained great respect for his judgment and learning.

David Atwater was a surgeon in General Wooster's brigade. He was killed in May, 1777, in the capture of Danbury by the British. The general was also killed in the engagement.

Edward Sutton was a surgeon in the northern department during the war, but died of dysentery, while in service, September 6, 1776.

Abriham Peet, a native of Bethlehem, Conn., after studying his profession, settled at Canaan, where he had a large practice. He died in the year 1786, at the age of 47.

Norman Morrison, a highly-educated physician, a native of Scotland, came to America and settled at Wethersfield, Conn., in 1740, but in a couple of years removed to Hartford, where he acquired a large practice, which he retained till the time of his death.

Joseph Perkins, a native of Norwich, Conn., an eminent physician and surgeon, practiced his profession in his native place, where he died 1794, aged 90. He was a graduate of Yale College in 1727. He was one of the most accomplished physicians and surgeons of his time, performing with success many daring and capital operations.

Oliver Wolcott, a native of Windsor, Mass., a graduate of Yale in 1747, was not only a good physician, but an ardent patriot during the Revolution, and held many important offices. He was a member of the Continental Congress and most of his life was devoted to public practice. He died December 1, 1797, aged 71.

Elihu Hubbard Smith was a native of Litchfield, Conn. He died of yellow fever in New York City, September 19, 1798. He was a graduate of Yale; studied medicine and settled in New York. Associated with Doctors Mitchell and Miller, he started the first medical journal in the United States, known as the New York Medical Repository.

Doctor Campbell was appointed surgeon's mate in Colonel Chapman's regiment of Connecticut volunteers in 1778 for coast-duty.

Dr. Elias Carrington, of Connecticut, was appointed by the legislature of that State, in October, 1776, as one of a board to examine applicants for the positions of surgeons and surgeon's mates in the Army.

Dr. Abel Castine, of Farrington, Conn., served as a surgeon during the Revolution. He died, at an advanced age, December 23, 1831.

Dr. Mason Fitch Cogswell, of Connecticut, was a surgeon in the Revolution. After the war he settled at Hartford. In 1803 he ligated the carotid artery.

John Dickinson was a physician, and died in Middleton, 1811, aged 82. He had held many offices of trust and was greatly esteemed.

Connecticut had many physicians of high literary and professional attainments and some who were noted for their large classes of private students. In this colony there are numerous examples of the clerical and medical professions combined in the same individual, and among the latest of this class was the Rev. Jared Eliot, who died in 1763.

Daniel Porter, celebrated as a bone-setter and general practitioner, was allowed an increase of salary in 1670, on the implied condition that he would "instruct some meet person in the art for which he was so distinguished."

The first medical degree granted on this continent is believed to be that conferred on Daniel Turner by Yale College, in 1720. As this degree was an honorary one and intended to be complimentary to Doctor Turner, who had been a liberal benefactor to the college, it was waggishly interpreted to signify *multum donavit*.

The medical department of Yale College was not regularly organized until 1813. This colony was quite celebrated, from its first settlement, for the number of its intelligent physicians, and next to Massachusetts advocated the most advanced theories of public education. Many of her physicians, from their superior acquirements and skill, occupied responsible positions under the government in colonial times, and in the Army during the Revolution; yet we do not find that they have contributed greatly to the literature of the profession.

Dr. John Ely established a hospital at Saybrook, in 1770, for the inoculation of the small-pox, (the first institution of the kind in the State,) which he conducted in an acceptable manner and with good success. He commanded a regiment of American troops during the revolutionary war. Died in 1800, aged 63.

Benjamin Gale, a native of Long Island, born 1715, published a treatise in 1750 on inoculation in America and advocated the preparation of the patients by a course of mercury. This was a meritorious work, and attracted attention from the profession in Europe, as well as in America. He published also in 1763 an essay on "The bite of the rattlesnake." He died at Killingworth, Conn., 1790.

Jared Eliot, a physician of distinction, was also a minister. He was a graduate of Yale College in 1706 and died April 22, 1763, aged 78

Josiah Rose, a native of Wethersfield, studied medicine in Boston and was a leading physician and surgeon of his day. He had five sons, who studied medicine and were surgeons in the revolutionary war. He died in 1786, aged 70.

Drs. John Bird, of Litchfield; Perry, sr., of Woodbury; James Potter, of New Fairfield; and William Jepson, of Hartford, were all prominent physicians in colonial times and about the close of the last century.

John Bulkley, a native of Colchester, combined the two professions of medicine and theology; was an exceedingly popular and influential person throughout the State, and held various offices of honor and trust. He died in 1754, aged 50.

Drs. John Simpson, John Noyes, John Watrous, and John Rose all held honorable positions as surgeons in the revolutionary army.

The Medical Society of the County of New Haven was instituted in 1784 and published a volume of cases and observations in 1788, which is among the earliest publications of the kind in our country.

John Osborne, a native of Massachusetts, was born in 1713. He was a distinguished physician, scholar, and poet, and was an alumnus of Harvard, in which institution he was proffered, but declined, a tutorship. Having studied medicine, he practiced at Middletown until his death, May 3, 1753.

Dr. John Osborne, his son, was born March 17, 1741, and, after practicing medicine at Middletown sixty years, died in June, 1825. He was in the medical department of the army in 1758, during the French and Indian war. He became a learned botanist and chemist.

Isaac Mosely graduated from Yale in 1762, studied medicine, and commenced practice at Glastonbury. His adherence to the British cause led to his removal to England. He was the author of a medical essay which attracted considerable professional attention.

Elizur Hale, of Glastonbury, graduated from Yale in 1742 and, having studied medicine, settled in his native town to practice. He died May 27, 1790, after having assiduously performed the duties of his calling forty-four years. He once represented that town in the general assembly.

His son, Elizur, also a practitioner, died in Glastonbury, December 6, 1796.

Elisha Phelps and Rev. Moses Bartlett, practitioners of medicine, resided at Portland from 1733 to 1766. The latter studied both medicine and theology with Dr. Phineas Fiske, of Haddam, himself a medico-theologian.

Dr. Aaron Roberts, of Cornwell, served throughout the revolutionary war as a surgeon and in 1783 removed to New Britain, where he died November 21, 1792, aged 62.

Moses Bartlett, son of the Rev. Moses Bartlett, also a physician, studied medicine with Dr. Benjamin Gale, of Willingworth, (now Clinton.) After completing his studies, he commenced practice in Portland. Died in 1810. His brother also studied under Dr. Gale, and located and practiced in Ashfield, Mass.

Asaph Coleman, a native of Colchester, was admitted to the practice of medicine by the Connecticut Medical Society in 1774. He located at Glastonbury, but, upon the breaking out of the Revolution, entered the Continental Army as surgeon to the Connecticut troops. He was several times elected representative to the general assembly. Died November 15, 1820, aged 73.

Dr. John Dickison, son of the Rev. Moses Dickison, of Norwalk, commenced practice at Wallingford, but by invitation of the selectmen removed to Middletown, where he acquired a good reputation and an extensive practice. As a representative, he occupied a seat in the legislature during the struggle for independence. After that period he relinquished the practice of medicine, and in 1793 was appointed judge of probate, and in 1796 judge of the county-court, both of which offices he retained until his death, in 1811, in the eighty-second year of his age.

Elisha Belcher was born in Preston, (now Lebanon,) in the year 1757, and, having received a good preliminary education, studied medicine. At the commencement of the revolutionary war he was appointed surgeon's mate in the Continental Army, and during that momentous struggle participated in many battles, and was finally promoted to a surgeoncy. He settled at Greenwich upon the cessation of hostilities, and not only did his reputation extend to the limits of his own county, but reached those of Westchester County, in the adjoining State, (New York.) He died in December, 1825, at the age of 69.

Eneas Munson was born at New Haven, June 24, 1734, and died June 16, 1826. He graduated at Yale in 1753 and was immediately appointed tutor in that institution. In 1755 he was appointed chaplain in the army, during the war with the French and Indians, but, soon leaving the military service, turned his attention to medicine, the study of which he began under Dr. John Darby, of East Hampton. Upon the completion of his studies, he settled at Bedford; served as a surgeon in the Continental Army, and was elected president of the Connecticut Medical Society; in 1760 moved to the town of his nativity, where he died.

Amos Skeele entered the Continental Army at the commencement of the war. Being wounded in the right arm, he left the military service and determined upon the study of medicine. He studied in Litchfield and afterward with Dr. Hastings, of Bethlehem. He began the practice at Haddam, but, after practicing in several places, finally settled at Chicopee, Mass., where he died, March 2, 1843, at the age of 93.

Robert Usher, a native of East Haddam, studied medicine with Dr. Huntingdon, of Windham, and began practice in 1762 at Chatham. In January, 1776, he entered the Continental Army as surgeon of Colonel Wadsworth's regiment, and served some time in that capacity, and died in the year 1820, aged 77.

CONNECTICUT SURGEONS IN THE REVOLUTION.

The following-named physicians of Connecticut served in their professional capacity in the American revolutionary army: David Adams, Isaac Brunson, Noah Coleman, Timothy Hosmer, Timothy Mather, John Noyes, John Rose, John Simpson, Justus Storrs, John R. Watrous, Samuel Lee of Windham, Aaron Roberts of New Britain, Albigeren Waldo of Windham, Laurett Hubbard of Hartford, and Isaac Smith of Greenwich.

Jared Potter and Witham Gould were commissioned, July 3, 1776, surgeon and surgeon's mate, respectively, of Col. William Douglas's regiment.

Surgeon David Holmes died March 20, 1779.

Thomas Skinner was commissioned in the medical department of the Army in 1775 or early in 1776.

The names of many other Connecticut physicians deserving of mention might be added if time and space permitted. No legislation that is deemed remarkable in its effect on the profession has been enacted in the State.[1]

---

[1] The following laws were enacted in Connecticut during the colonial government: An act providing in case of contagious sickness, enacted 1711, Stat. Conn., ed. 1715, p. 160; An act to prevent the small-pox being spread in this colony by pedlars, hawkers, and petty chapmen, enacted 1722, Stat. Conn., p. 270; Physicians and chirurgeons to be exempt from performing military duty, enacted 1722, Stat. Conn., p. 78, act regulating militia; Physicians and chirurgeons to be taxed and rated as others, enacted 1722, Stat. Conn., p. 282; An act amending the act of 1711, enacted 1728, Stat. Conn., p. 352; An act providing in all cases of contagious sickness, enacted 1729, Stat. Conn., 1750, p. 225; An act providing in case of infectious diseases, enacted 1732, Stat. Conn., p. 391; An act additive to the act of 1729, requiring that all goods coming from infected places be aired before exposure for sale, enacted 1752, Stat. Conn., ed. 1769, p. 265; An act additive to the foregoing, providing for vessels coming from infected ports, enacted

EARLY PHYSICIANS IN RHODE ISLAND.

Dr. John Clark, formerly a physician of London, was one of the founders of Rhode Island. He originally settled in Boston, but was banished, and, with Roger Williams, sought an asylum in the new region to the south. When the church in that colony was organized, in 1644, he was appointed pastor and in 1649 was made assistant treasurer of the colony. He died at Newport, April 20, 1676, at the age of 67 years, leaving a reputation unsurpassed for purity of life.

Dr. William Hunter, a Scotchman by birth, and a member of the distinguished family of that name, came to the colony of Rhode Island in 1752. He lectured upon anatomy and surgery in the years 1755 and 1756, not only to medical men and students, but to the literary gentlemen of the city of Newport. He also served as a surgeon in the French and Indian war. An oil-portrait of the doctor is in the possession of Mr. Hunter, of the State-Department, in Washington, who is a lineal descendant of the doctor.

Dr. Haliburton, a contemporary of Dr. Hunter, was his rival in talent and professional ability.

Dr. Bowen, a physician of eminence, resided in Rhode Island, and enjoyed the confidence of the people as early as 1640, probably coming in with the second party from Massachusetts.

In 1663, Capt. John Cranston was licensed by the general court " to administer physicke and practice chirurgerie," and had conferred upon him the degree of M. D., in the following words: "And is by this court styled doctor of physick and chirurgery by the authority of this the general assembly of this colony," (Rhode Island.) This may be claimed, perhaps, to be the first medical degree conferred in America.

Pierre Ayrault, a French refugee, who settled in the colony in the year 1686, was a practitioner of physic.

Drs. John Bret and Thomas Moffatt enjoyed medical reputation as early as 1751. The estate of the latter, on account of his British proclivities, was forfeited in 1775.

Dr. Ephraim Bowen, the originator of the order known as the Daughters of Liberty, was practicing his profession in Rhode Island in 1766.

Jabez Brown, a native of Seekonk, R. I., was practicing medicine at Providence as early as the year 1700.

A son of his, Jabez Brown, and Benjamin West, practitioners of medicine, assisted Joseph Brown, of Providence, in determining the latitude and longitude of that town during the transit of Venus, in 1769.

John Mawney, a medical student, rendered professional services to

---

1756, Stat. Conn., 1769, p. 281; An act additive to the same, regulating inoculation, enacted 1760, Stat. Conn., 1769, p. 298; An act additive to the same, concerning inoculation, enacted 1760, Stat. Conn., 1769, p. 300; An act additive to the same, concerning inoculation, enacted 1761, Stat. Conn., ed. 1769, p. 302; An act reviving the original act of 1729, with all its additions, enacted 1769, Stat. Conn., ed. 1769, pp. 305–344; An act for the suppression of mountebanks, (dealers in quack medicines,) enacted 1773, Stat. Conn., p. 389.

Duddington, who was wounded in an expedition commanded by Capt. Abraham Whipple, in 1772.

Jonathan Arnold, a physician of Providence, was a deputy to the Continental Congress in 1776, a strenuous opponent of the claims of the King. In 1782 he sustained Mr. Howell in his protest against the infringement by Congress upon the rights of the State and was re-elected to Congress in the following year.

Isaac Senter, a native of Londonderry, N. H., was studying medicine at Newport when the news of the battle of Lexington reached him; and, filled with patriotic ardor, he immediately joined the Rhode Island troops as surgeon of a regiment. He accompanied the secret expedition of General Arnold to Quebec in 1775 and kept a private journal of the march. He was taken prisoner, but was afterward released. In 1779 he retired from the Army, and commenced practice at Cranston, and subsequently removed to Newport. From the former town he was sent as a representative to the general assembly. He was appointed physician and surgeon-general of the State, and contributed several papers to the literature of medicine; one, An Account of a Singular Case of Ischuria, published in 18th vol. Memoirs of the Medical Society of London. He died in 1799.

Richard Bowen was a physician in practice at Seekonk, R. I., as early as 1680. His residence was in proximity to Providence and he visited the sick of that place.

Norbert Felician Vigneron was a native of France; was an educated physician; emigrated with his family and settled in Newport, R. I., in 1690; pursued the practice of his profession until the time of his death, 1794, aged 95. His son, Charles Antonius Vigneron, also studied mediicine, and practiced in Rhode Island and in New York, where he died of small-pox in 1772. A son of the late Stephen Vigneron was a surgeon in the United States Navy during the revolutionary war, but was lost at sea.

Thomas Redman, a native of England, was educated to the profession of medicine. In 1680 he settled to practice at Newport and was a popular physician. He died in 1727, aged 80.

Joseph Hewes, a surgeon during the revolutionary war, practiced at Providence. He was the preceptor of many young men who rose to eminence in the profession. He died September 30, 1796, aged 82.

Sylvester Gardner, a native of South Kingston, R. I., died at Newport, August 8, 1796, aged 69. He had received a good classical and medical education. He settled to practice in Boston, where he acquired wealth. On the breaking out of the war he sided with Great Britain, and abandoned all his property. After peace was restored he returned to Newport and again engaged in practice with success and reputation.

Daniel Lee, a physician of some note, died of yellow fever at Westerly, Washington County, R. I., September 10, 1798, aged 41.

William Bradford, a native of Plympton, Mass., was an accomplished physician, and practiced for half a century in Bristol, R. I., where he died July 6, 1808, aged 79. He was a lineal descendant of Hon. W. Bradford, one of the Pilgrim Fathers. In addition to his practice as a physician he studied law, and for years was one of the leading men in the State and an ardent patriot in the Revolution.

Ephraim Bowen, qualifying himself for the practice of medicine, settled in Providence, R. I., where he spent a long and useful life. He died October 12, 1812, aged 96.

Daniel Peck Whipple, a native of Rhode Island, was a surgeon in the revolutionary war, serving part of the time in the Navy and part in the Army. He died in Cumberland, R. I., May 19, 1814.

Amos Throop, a native of Connecticut, studied medicine and settled in Providence, R. I., and engaged actively in practice until his death, April, 1814, aged 76. He was the first physician in Providence who set up as an obstetrician. He was the first president of the Rhode Island Medical Society. He also filled offices of honor and trust in the State.

Peter Turner, a native of Newark, N. J., at the commencement of the war was commissioned surgeon of Colonel Green's Rhode Island regiment. He had settled to practice at Greenwich. After the war he returned to his practice, which was large and lucrative to the time of his death, which occurred February 14, 1822, at the age of 71.

Pardon Bowen was born in Providence, R. I. He was a physician of great eminence; was a graduate of Rhode Island College (now Brown University) and a surgeon in the Revolution. He was through life a close observer and wrote some valuable papers, one particularly on yellow fever. He died at Norwich, R. I., aged 69.

Samuel Tenny, a native of Byfield, Mass., was educated at Harvard College, and studied medicine. He rendered medical services at the battle of Bunker Hill and served as a surgeon in the American Army in Colonel Israel's Rhode Island troops. At the close of the war he settled at Exeter, N. H., where he remained until his death, in the year 1816. He was judge of probate for many years and was elected to the United States Congress in 1800, and served to 1807. His death occurred in 1816.

The following gentlemen served as surgeons in the Rhode Island provincial troops during the French and Indian war: John Bass, (who was also a chaplain,) Benjamin Brown, Thomas Monroe, Christopher Nichols, and Thomas Rodman.

John Bartlett, Nicholas N. Bogart, John Chace, Joseph Rhodes, Ebenezer Richmond, Levi Wheaton, John Parish, and Joseph Bowen, who served as surgeons in the American revolutionary army, were all residents of this State.[1]

---

[1] The only act passed by the colonial government of Rhode Island of interest in our present inquiry is one entitled "An act to prevent the spreading of the small-pox and other contagious diseases in this State," which was enacted in 1743 and revived and revised in 1748.—(Stat. R. I., ed. 1798, fol. 335.)

MEDICAL SCIENCE ELSEWHERE.

Going farther southward, we find in New York the earliest recorded instance of a demonstration from the cadaver for the instruction of students.

In 1750 Drs. Middleton and Bard injected and dissected the body of an executed criminal before their students. In the same city Dr. Samuel Clossy, a Dublin graduate, began courses of lectures on anatomy.

In the Jerseys, Thos. Wood, surgeon, in 1752, advertised through the New York press "A course on osteology and myology in the city of New Brunswick," of about one month's continuance, to be followed, if proper encouragement was given, by a "Course on angiology and neurology," and conclude with performing all the operations on the dead body.

EARLY PHYSICIANS IN NEW JERSEY.

The earliest physician in New Jersey of whom we have any record was Abraham Peirson, also a minister of the gospel, a native of Yorkshire, England. He graduated at Cambridge in 1632 and immigrated to Boston in 1639. He removed to Southampton, R. I., and subsequently, in 1667, to Newark, N. J., and was the first minister of that town. He died August 7, 1678.

Dr. Jonathan Dickinson, a native of Hatfield, Mass., was the first president of Princeton College (formerly the college of New Jersey) and the first pastor of the Presbyterian church of Elizabeth. He was also a practicing physician of considerable repute during the first forty years of the last century. He died October 7, 1747, aged 59 years.

William Turner studied medicine with Dr. N. T. Pinquerou, a Frenchman from the province D'Artois, who had settled in Newport, R. I., in 1690, and, having finished his studies, removed to Newark, where he practiced his profession probably to the time of his death, which occurred subsequently to 1750.

Daniel Cox was a physician in extensive practice in London, but it is doubtful if he practiced in America. In 1690 he purchased the greater part of West Jersey, and was constituted governor of his grant. He appointed a deputy, however, rather than relinquish his professional business, and eventually sold his right to Sir Thomas Lane.

Dr. Jacob Arents, a Hollander, was naturalized in the year 1716, and practiced medicine in Newark from that time until the year 1750.

John Rockhill, a member of the Society of Friends, was born in Burlington County, March 22, 1726, and studied medicine under Dr. Thomas Cadwallader, of Philadelphia. He settled at Pittstown in 1748 and enjoyed a remunerative and extensive practice for nearly fifty years. He died April 7, 1798.

Dr. John Gerard Shults practiced medicine in Essex County as early as 1730. He is supposed to have been a native of Holland, who came originally to New York, but subsequently removed to New Jersey.

Elijah Bowen, the earliest practitioner of medicine in Cumberland

County, began practice at Shiloh in 1730 and continued until his death, which took place September 26, 1773, at an advanced age. Tradition says that he used vegetable-remedies only.

Dr. Elijah Bowen, jr., son of the preceding, was born in Cohansey in 1714, and died, December 21, 1765, at the age of 51, at Hopewell. Like his father, he obtained his remedies from the vegetable-kingdom.

Dr. Seth Ward, a native of Connecticut, came to Greenwich in 1760 and practiced until his death, which occurred, February 27, 1774, at the age of 38 years.

Gersham Craven graduated at Princeton College in 1765 and, having attended medical lectures at the University of Pennsylvania, located at Rangoes, in 1771, where he became popular and very successful in his profession. He died, May 3, 1819, at the age of 75 years.

Jonathan Elmer was born at Cedarville, November 29, 1745, and, having finished his preliminary education, commenced the study of medicine with Dr. John Morgan, of Philadelphia. He attended the first course of lectures delivered in the medical school of the University of Pennsylvania, received the degree of M. B. in 1768, and commenced the practice of his profession at Roadstown, but afterward removed to Bridgeton. In 1771 the degree of M. B. was conferred upon him. In 1772 he was appointed sheriff of Cumberland County, but was deposed for expressed hostility to British encroachments. He was also, respectively, a delegate to the Provincial and Continental Congresses, an officer in the American revolutionary army, clerk of the county, judge of probate, a United States Representative, and Senator. He died September 3, 1814, aged 72 years.

Dr. Robert Halsted was born September 13, 1746, and died at Elizabethtown in 1825. He was an able physician, and having rendered services to the continental soldiers he was imprisoned by the British on the information of a tory neighbor.

Thomas Ewing, the great grandson of Finley Ewing, an Irish patriot who had been presented with a sword by King William for bravery at the battle of the Boyne, was born at Greenwich, September 13, 1748. He received a classical education and began the study of medicine with Dr. Samuel Ward, of Greenwich; but upon completing his studies removed to Cape May, where he commenced practice. After the death of his preceptor he returned to his native town and practiced there until his death, which was caused by consumption, October 7, 1782. He received an appointment as surgeon, and afterward as major, in the American Army and served during the revolutionary war.

Dr. Deancy practiced medicine at Newark as early as the year 1748.

Dr. George Andrew Veisselius, a native of Germany or Holland, immigrated to this country in 1749 and located himself at Three Bridges, where he afterward married. He was a skillful and successful physician. After his death, in 1767, his wife, an amiable and intelligent woman, was frequently called upon by her neighbors for medical advice.

Dr. Uzal Johnson, born April 17, 1751, died May 22, 1827, was a practitioner of medicine. He was elected to the Provincial Congress in 1775, but declined the position and entered the British army. Being lame, he always rode in a small-wheeled carriage, upon the panels of which was emblazoned the motto "Non nunquam paratus."

Dr. Caleb Halsted, son of Dr. Robert Halsted, was born in Elizabeth, September 5, 1752, and died, August 18, 1827, at the age of 75 years. He was a leading physician of his day and rendered professional services to many French families of the nobility who settled in and about Elizabeth. When General Marquis de La Fayette came to this country, in 1825, he paid a visit to the doctor, then in his seventy-third year.

Ebenezer Elmer, brother of Dr. Jonathan Elmer, was born at Cedarville, in 1752. Having received a classical education, he studied medicine, but before completing his course he entered the Army as an ensign, which position, however, he resigned, in 1777, for an appointment in the medical department of the Army. In 1789 he was elected speaker of the general assembly, and afterward a Representative in the United States Congress, and was also a general of militia during the war of 1812. He held at various times during his life numerous State- and Federal offices and died, October 18, 1843, in the ninety-first year of his age.

John Darby, a Presbyterian divine and also a physician, practiced medicine at Parsippany as early as 1750. He died in 1805, aged 80 years. His son, Henry White Darby, having graduated at one of the eastern colleges, studied medicine and practiced at Parsippany, where he died, in December, 1806, at the age of 48 years.

John Hanna, a native of Ireland, graduated at Princeton College in 1755, studied medicine and theology, and was appointed pastor of the Presbyterian church at Bethlehem, but subsequently at Kingwood, Pittstown, and Alexandria, at which latter place he died, November 4, 1801, at the age of 70 years. He maintained a good reputation as a physician.

Lewis Howell, a twin brother of Richard Howell, governor of New Jersey, was born, October 25, 1754, in Delaware, and removed to Cumberland County, New Jersey, with his parents, where he shortly afterward commenced the study of medicine with Dr. Jonathan Elmer. In 1777, having completed his studies, he was commissioned a surgeon in the Continental Army. On the day before the battle of Monmouth, he was taken suddenly ill, at Monmouth Court-House, and died on the day of the battle.

Dr. John Condict, born at Orange, July 15, 1755, was a practitioner with large professional business. He was a surgeon and afterward a colonel in the Continental Army, and also a member of the New Jersey legislature.

George Campbell was born in Tyrone County, Ireland, August 15, 1758, graduated at the University of Dublin, and studied medicine under Doctor

McFarlin. He immigrated to America while the revolutionary war was in progress and entered the American Army as a surgeon. At the close of the war he commenced practice in Franklin and soon acquired a large and remunerative business. In 1818 he was stricken with paralysis, which caused his death in the sixtieth year of his age.

Isaac Morse, a Quaker, descended of noble ancestry, was born at Rahway, August 5, 1758, and died at Elizabeth, July 23, 1825. He was a student under Dr. William Barnet. He was very popular as a citizen and his reputation as a physician was good.

Dr. James Johnson, a native of England, practiced at Roadstown previously to the time of his death, which occurred, May 25, 1759, in the fifty-third year of his age. He is said to have married the daughter of an Indian chief.

Samuel Moore Shute was born in Cumberland County, in 1762, and, although but 14 years old at the breaking-out of the Revolution, his name appears upon the records of the revolutionary war as an officer in the Army. After leaving the military service he entered the office of Dr. Jonathan Elmer as a student and on the completion of his studies settled in Bridgeton, where he died August 30, 1816, at the age of 54 years. He was one of the leading practitioners of the town and was appointed surrogate of Cumberland County by the governor of that State.

Dr. Bernard Budd was one of the fourteen original founders of the New Jersey Medical Society, which was organized in 1766 and incorporated in 1790. He was a surgeon in the revolutionary war, and his reputation as such was second to none of that period. His son, John C. Budd, was born May 26, 1762, at Morristown, and died January 12, 1845. His medical studies were prosecuted under Dr. John Condict, of Orange, and he was a skillful practitioner.

Oliver Barnet practiced medicine at New Germantown as early as 1765. He acquired an excellent reputation as a physician, but his patients often complained of his excessive charges. He died December 25, 1809, in the sixty-sixth year of his age, after having amassed a fortune of over eighty thousand dollars from his professional business.

John D. Williams was born November 5, 1765, studied medicine with Dr. Daniel Barret, and commenced practice at Connecticut Farms. He married a sister of the elder Governor Pennington and was appointed a magistrate for the county of Essex. He was the first president of the New Jersey Medical Society and died January 5, 1826.

The first resident physician of Flemington was Dr. Creed, who practiced there as early as 1765.

Aaron Forman, a practitioner of medicine, was born February 4, 1745, in Wales, and, having immigrated to this country, died in Hunterdon County, January 11, 1805. He was a prominent physician and surgeon, careful of his reputation and proud of his profession.

Dr. Samuel Johnson, a practitioner of medicine at Newark, died August 7, 1770, aged 36.

Dr. Paul Michlau, a physician of Elizabeth, was enrolled a member of the State Medical Society in 1772.

Dr. Ichabod Burnet, a native of Scotland, practiced medicine in Elizabeth. He died in 1774, at the age of 90. His son, William Burnet, was born December 2, 1730, and joined the American Continental Army (at the commencement of the struggle for independence) as a surgeon and in the fall of 1775 was appointed surgeon of the United States Hospital. In 1776 he was chosen to the Continental Congress and later was constituted physician and surgeon-general of the eastern district, which latter position he held until the close of the war. He died in 1791, aged 61.

Dr. John Griffith was practicing physic at Rahway at the time of the organization of the medical society and was president of it in 1790.

Robert Patterson, a native of Ireland, kept a store in Bridgeton in 1773, but, abandoning the mercantile business, commenced the study of medicine and after completing a course of studies entered the Army as an assistant surgeon. Cumberland County became the theater of his professional labors after his leaving the Army. In 1779 he was appointed professor of mathematics in the University of Pennsylvania; later, Director of the Mint, by President Jefferson; and finally, in 1819, was elected president of the American Philosophical Society. Died in 1824, aged 82.

Mathias Peirson was born in Orange, June 20, 1734, and spent his life in the practice of medicine in that town. He died May 9, 1808, aged 74. Descendants of his, bearing the same name, still adorn the profession in New Jersey and other States of the Union.

Dr. Edward Pigot was one of the earliest physicians of Essex County.

Drs. William Barnet, William Burnel, Jabez Campfield, Moses G. Elmer, Jacob Harris, Otto Bodo, Benjamin Stockton, and Garrett Tunison were surgeons to the New Jersey troops in the Continental Army.

FORMATION OF MEDICAL SOCIETIES.

In New Jersey a general or State medical society was organized on the voluntary principle in 1766 and was incorporated by the State in 1790. This was the second, if not the first, medical association of the country, and the only one that has survived which is known to have preserved records and transactions that antedate the Revolution.

Their desire to elevate the standard of medical education is evident, as rules were prescribed to its members at an early day in reference to receiving medical apprentices under their charge.[1]

Its regulations provided that "The apprentice must be refused unless

---

[1] The following-named gentlemen were the founders and original members of the New Jersey Medical Society, which was established July 20, 1766:

Robert McKean, Christopher Manlove, John Cockran, Moses Bloomfield, James Gilliland, William Burnet, Jonathan Dayton, Thomas Wiggins, William Adams, Bernard Budd, Lawrence van Derveer, John Griffith, Isaac Harris, Joseph Sacket.

he has a competent knowledge of Latin and some acquaintance with the rudiments of Greek and will serve not less than four years, one of which may be spent abroad, and pay one hundred pounds, proclamation-money, as apprentice-fee." The general assembly of New Jersey, in 1772, for the first time, passed a law regulating the practice of medicine in the province, requiring all practitioners of medicine to be examined and licensed under the direction of at least two of the judges of the supreme court, upon due examination of his learning and skill in physic and surgery. This law followed closely the stipulations and preserved the spirit of an act passed in the colony of New York, in 1760, for the regulation of practice in the city of New York, and seems to have exercised a good influence.

John Morgan, immediately on his return to Philadelphia, in 1765, was instrumental in organizing a medical society, called the Philadelphia Medical Society, which was the first in Pennsylvania. An American medical society was formed in Philadelphia in 1783, of which Dr. William Shippen was president and Dr. Henry Stuber secretary. I have seen no record of its labors.

The College of Physicians of Philadelphia was established in 1787, and has always been the supporter of high ethics in the profession, and has done much in this regard. It has published numerous volumes of contributions to the literature of the profession.[1] The Delaware State Medical Society was organized in 1776. The Medical Society of Massachusetts was formed in 1781. The South Carolina Medical Association was founded 1789 and chartered by the legislature in 1794. The Medical Society of New Hampshire was formed in 1791; the Medical Society of Connecticut in 1784. The Medical and Chirurgical Faculty of the State of Maryland was incorporated in 1799.

EARLY PHYSICIANS IN PENNSYLVANIA.

Thomas Wynne,[2] a Welsh physician, and his brother, also a physician, settled in Philadelphia in 1682. They came with William Penn in the Welcome.[3] He had a taste for public affairs and was elected member of the provincial assembly.

Griffith Owen was an English physician and among the early followers of Penn. He amputated an arm in 1699 at Chester.[4] He died in 1717, aged 70. He left a son, a physician in practice.

John Goodson, also an English physician, was in active practice in Philadelphia as early as 1700.

Dr. Hodgson was also practicing at the same period in Philadelphia.

Edward Jones, a physician of note, arrived in Philadelphia, June 13,

---

[1] Carson's History of the University of Pennsylvania, p. 222.
[2] Proud's History of Pennsylvania.
[3] Carson's History of the University of Pennsylvania.
[4] Journal of the life of Thomas Story, p. 245.

1682, and was probably one of the original immigrants to this colony. He was a son-in-law of Dr. Thomas Wynne.

Evan Jones, a brother of the former, came to the colony about the same time and was a prominent physician.

Christopher Witt, a physician of extensive learning, came to Philadelphia in 1704. He was eccentric in his habits and the vulgar suspected him of being a conjurer. He died in 1769, aged 90.

John Kearsley, an English physician, arrived in the colony about 1711 and Thomas Graeme in 1719. Graeme was a highly-educated physician and distinguished citizen. He was a popular member of the assembly and a champion of the rights of the people. He contributed largely to the building of Christ Church and left a valuable estate to endow a widows' hospital. He died in 1772, aged 82.

Lloyd Zachary, as early as 1720, was in practice.

Owen Griffith, a young man of promise in the profession, died in 1731, aged 25.

William Gardiner, a native of Germany, having been educated as a physician, immigrated to America and settled in Lancaster, Pa., where he practiced with reputation until he died in 1756, aged 45.

Phineas Bond, M. D., a native of Maryland, was regularly educated to medicine in Europe. He was a brother of Dr. Thomas Bond and settled to practice in Philadelphia, where he rose to eminence and enjoyed the confidence of the whole country. He died in 1773, aged 56.

Cadwallader Evans was born in Philadelphia; studied medicine and graduated in England. He settled in his native place. In 1759 he was one of the physicians to the Pennsylvania Hospital, a position which he held with ability to the time of his death in 1773, aged 57.

John Bartram, a native of Delaware County, Pa., and a son of a physician of the same name, who was killed by the Whitoc Indians in North Carolina, studied medicine and settled in Philadelphia. He was an eminent botanist, and explained and explored almost all the Atlantic coast and settled parts of North America. His contributions to the science of botany and natural history were numerous and valuable. He died in Philadelphia in 1777.

Thomas Cadwallader, M. D., was a native of Philadelphia; received a good classical education; studied medicine with Dr. Evan Jones; he also attended lectures in Europe. He was the first physician in Philadelphia to make dissections and subsequently assisted Dr. Shippen in his lectures before his class. He was among the earliest contributors to medical literature in America. In 1745 he published an "Essay on the iliac passion." He was one of the first corps of physicians appointed to the Pennsylvania Hospital in 1751. He was greatly beloved by all. He died November 14, 1779, aged 72.

Adam Simon Kuhn, a native of Germany, was brought when a child with his father, who settled as a farmer near Lancaster, Pa., in 1733. Having studied medicine he practiced in Lancaster. He was a good classical scholar and a man of fine natural abilities and a great supporter of public education. He died July 23, 1780, aged 66.

George Glentworth, a native of Philadelphia, was educated to the medical profession in Europe, graduating in Edinburgh, in 1755. In 1758 he was a junior surgeon in the British army. He took sides with the patriots in the Revolution and was commissioned surgeon in the American Army and assisted in extracting the ball that wounded General Lafayette at Brandywine. He died in 1792.

James Hutchinson, a practitioner of Bucks County, Pa., died of yellow fever in Philadelphia in 1793. He was a physician of superior acquirements and an excellent chemist. He was a surgeon in the revolutionary war. He held at one time the chair of chemistry and materia medica in the University of Pennsylvania.

Samuel Preston Moore was a native of Philadelphia and son of Dr. Nicholas Moore, president of the True Society of Traders, who came to America with William Penn. He studied medicine with his father, was a good physician and of good business-habits. He inherited large landed property from his father and was treasurer of the general assembly. He was one of the early contributors and one of the first physicians appointed to attend the Pennsylvania Hospital. He died in Philadelphia, July 15, 1785, aged 76.

David Jackson, a surgeon of the revolutionary war, died in Philadelphia September 17, 1801. He was the father of Prof. Samuel Jackson, of the University of Pennsylvania.

William Irvine, a native of Ireland, was educated to the medical profession and was for some years a surgeon in the British navy. Having resigned, he immigrated to America and settled at Carlisle, Pa. On the breaking-out of the Revolution he took part with the colonies and filled numerous important posts as surgeon and as commander, with a rank as high as major-general. He was elected to and served in Congress from 1786 to 1788. He died July 30, 1804, in Philadelphia.

Absalom Baird, a native of Pennsylvania, was a surgeon in the Revolution. He died near Pittsburg, Pa., October 27, 1805.

John Redman, a native of Pennsylvania, was educated to the profession of medicine, and graduated at Leyden in 1748. He was one of the first corps of physicians in 1751 appointed to the Pennsylvania Hospital, a post he held until 1780. He possessed fine literary acquirements, was a close reasoner and a most excellent and judicious practitioner, and exercised great influence upon the profession in Philadelphia. In 1759 he published a defense of inoculation and advised the use of mercury in preserving the patient. He was the first president of the College of Physicians. He died March 19, 1807.

John Wilkins, a native of Pennsylvania, was a surgeon in Col. William Butler's regiment in the Revolution. He was subsequently in the commissary-department of the United States Army, and was therefore better known as General Wilkins. He died in Western Pennsylvania in April, 1816.

Nathaniel Bedford was a well-educated English surgeon who ;settled in Pittsburg as early as 1783, probably the first educated physician to settle there. He practiced there with success during the remainder of his life and died about 1815. Dr. Peter Moway was his successor in practice.

George Logan was a native of Pennsylvania and grandson of James Logan. He received a good classical education and then studied medicine and received the degree of M. D. from the University of Edinburgh in 1779. He settled to practice at his homestead, "Stouton," in Philadelphia, and combined agriculture with the duties of his profession. He was popular both as a physician and as a citizen; was sent several times to the State-legislature. In 1798 he went to France for the sole purpose of endeavoring to prevent hostilities between that nation and the United States, and no doubt accomplished some useful purpose to that end. He was United States Senator from Pennsylvania from 1801 to 1807. He was a member of the Philosophical Society and other local associations. He died April 9, 1821.

Stephen Munroe was one of the early physicians in Fayette County, Pa. He practiced in Sutton, where he died, September 9, 1826, at an advanced age.

John Morgan, M. D., was born at Philadelphia in 1735 and in 1757 received the first literary honors conferred by the College of Philadelphia. Previous to his graduation he commenced the study of medicine with Dr. John Redman, and having completed his studies entered the Provincial Army as a lieutenant and surgeon in the war with the French and Indians; left the Army in 1760 and sailed to Europe for the purpose of finishing his medical education. In 1762 the degree of M. D. was conferred on him by the University of Edinburgh. He went to Paris, made an extensive tour of Europe, and was elected member of several learned societies. After his return home he began practice, was the co-founder with Dr. Shippen of the medical department of the College of Philadelphia, and was elected professor of theory and practice.

At the commencement of the Revolution he was appointed by Congress director-general and physician-in-chief to the hospital of the American Army, but was afterward removed on groundless charges preferred against him. He died, October 15, 1789, in his fifty-fourth year.

His publications were "A discourse on the institution of medical schools in Philadelphia," 1765 ; " A prize essay on the reciprocal advantages of a perpetual union between Great Britain and her colonies ;" "A recommendation of inoculation," in 1776; " Vindication of his public character as director of the general hospital," 1777 ; and a number of papers in the Transactions of the American Philosophical Society, an institution of which he was one of the founders.

Dr. Prentice, of Carlisle, was a practitioner of medicine and surgery, and rendered professional aid to the wounded of the English army after an engagement with the French and Indians, in April, 1756. Dr. Jamison, surgeon of the provincial troops, participating in the battle, was missing.

Adam Kuhn, son of Dr. Adam Simon Kuhn, was born in Germantown, November 17, 1741, and died July 5, 1817, at the age of 76. He received a classical education and studied medicine with his father until the year 1761, when he sailed for Europe and entered the University of Upsal, under the celebrated Linnæus. After studying there one year, he matriculated at Edinburgh, whence he obtained his degree, June 12, 1767. On his return to Philadelphia, the following year, he was appointed professor of materia medica in the College of Philadelphia and, subsequently, professor of the theory and practice of medicine in the University of Pennsylvania. He was on the committee of safety and board of examining surgeons and was director-general of the hospital for New Jersey troops. He was a member of nearly all the American scientific societies then in existence.

Benjamin Rush was born on his father's plantation, fourteen miles from Philadelphia, December 24, 1745, and died at Philadelphia, April 18, 1813, at the age of 68. He graduated at Princeton before he completed his fifteenth year and studied medicine with Dr. John Redman and William Shippen, to the former of whom he was apprenticed for six years. In 1766 he sailed for Europe, matriculated at Edinburgh, and graduated in 1768 with the degree of doctor of medicine. At different times he filled various chairs in the University of Pennsylvania; also, in the College of Philadelphia; was physician-general of the hospital of the middle military department; was a member of the convention for draughting the Constitution of the United States, and for the last fourteen years of his life was treasurer of the United States Mint. He was a member of the Continental Congress in 1776, and as such his name is attached to the Declaration of Independence. He was a voluminous and varied writer, his works treating upon nearly all branches of science. He had great power for original observation and has left the impress of his genius on the theory of medicine in the United States which the lapse of a hundred years has not effaced.

The first regularly-bred physician of Dauphin County was Dr. McLelland, of Greencastle. He was very successful in his practice, which extended over an area of sixty miles.

Dr. William Shippen, sr., was the son of Edward Shippen, the immigrant. He studied medicine and practiced with success and reputation in Philadelphia during a long life. He was one of the founders of the College of New Jersey. He was one of the vice-presidents of the Philosophical Society and one of the first physicians of the Pennsylvania Hospital. He also served a term as a member of Congress. He died November 4, 1801, aged 89.

Dr. William Shippen, son of the above-named, of Philadelphia, was born in 1736 and graduated at the College of New Jersey in 1754. He spent three years after his graduation in the study of medicine with his father, and at the age of 21 sailed for Europe, entered at Edinburgh, received the doctorate degree, and returned to his native city in the year 1762. On his return to Philadelphia he commenced a course of medical lectures on anatomy in 1762. He occupied at different times several chairs in the College of Philadelphia and University of Pennsylvania. In 1776 he entered the medical department of the Continental Army as Medical Director-General, but resigned, in 1781, that position, in order to devote his undivided attention to the medical school, of which he was one of the faculty. His death, which occurred July 11, 1808, was hastened, it is believed, by grief at the death of his only son.

Dr. Caspar Wistar, a member of the Society of Friends, was born in Philadelphia, September 13, 1761. At the battle of Germantown, although prohibited from participating on account of religious scruples, he assisted the American surgeons in attending the wounded, which was probably the foundation of his future avocation. He studied medicine with Drs. John Jones and John Redman and graduated at the University of Pennsylvania in 1782 with the degree of M. B. In 1783 he sailed for Europe, and, having entered the University of Edinburgh, the degree of M. D. was conferred upon him in 1786. While in Great Britain he was, for two successive years, president of the Royal Medical Society of Edinburgh and president of the Society for the Investigation of Natural History. On his return to America he was appointed physician to the Philadelphia Dispensary. Was a member of nearly all the learned societies in the city and was elected to various professorships in the University of Pennsylvania. Died of typhus-fever, January 22, 1818.

PENNSYLVANIA SURGEONS IN THE REVOLUTION.

The following gentlemen of the medical faculty of Pennsylvania served in the American Continental Army as surgeons:

William Adams, Richard Allison, Absalom Baird, Reading Beatty, Thomas Bond, James Brown, Andrew Caldwell, James Davidson, Robert Harris, Robert Johnson, Andrew Ladley, William Magaw, Hugh Martin, Matthew Mans, Thomas McCalla, Samuel A. McCoffrey, Alexander McCosky, John McDowell, Robert Nicholson, Peter J. Peres, Samuel Platt, John Rogne, John A. Saple, William Smith, George Stevenson, Alexander Stewart, Christopher Taylor, Joseph Thompson, Garrett van Wagenner, Robert Wharry, John Wilkins, and Aaron Woodruff.[1]

---

[1] I find upon examination that the following-entitled laws were enacted in Pennsylvania during the period of the colonial government: An act to prevent sickly vessels coming into this government, enacted 1700, Stat. Pa., ed. 1775, fol. 12; An act vesting the Province Island, and the buildings thereon erected and to be erected, in trustees, and for providing an hospital for such sick passengers as shall be imported into this province, and to prevent the spreading of infectious distempers, enacted

Christian Reineck was killed at Paoli, Pa., in the service. Abel Morgan, a surgeon of the Revolution, died July, 1795. Robert Nicholson, of York County, Pa., a surgeon in the Revolution, died August 15, 1798. Charles McCarter, a surgeon of the Revolution, died in 1800. John Rogers, a surgeon, died in New York, July 29, 1833. Samuel Sackett, a surgeon, died in Fayette County, Pa., February 13, 1833.

Surgeons John Lockman and Henry Malcolm died in Philadelphia County, the former August 16, 1819, and the latter April 18, 1831.

Surgeon John Ramsey died November 4, 1776. Surgeon Christopher Reinick died September 21, 1777. Dr. John R. B. Rogers died in New York, January 29, 1833. He had served in the revolutionary war as a surgeon in the Pennsylvania troops.

In Pennsylvania dissections were made for the benefit of the physicians of Philadelphia, if not anterior to, certainly as early as, 1751, by Dr. Thomas Cadwallader, a native of that city, who completed his professional studies in European schools.

He published in 1740 an essay on the "Dry gripes, with the method of curing the cruel distemper;" printed and sold by B. Franklin, Philadelphia, 1745. It is probable that the doctor's early dissections were to further illustrate his investigations in these diseases and that they therefore antedate all the autopsies for pathological studies in the United States.

Thomas Bond was a native of Maryland. He studied medicine with Dr. Hamilton, of Annapolis. Having acquired proficiency in his profession, he settled to practice in Philadelphia in 1734. He was one of the founders of the college which preceded the University of Pennsylvania. Dr. Franklin gave him credit for originating the project for the Pennsylvania Hospital. He was large-minded, well-informed, and painstaking in everything that related to his profession, and he published in 1754, in the London Medical Observations and Enquiries, an account of a "worm bred in the liver," and in 1759 a paper on the use of "bark" in scrofulous cases. Dr. Cadwallader Evans published in 1754, in Medical Observations and Enquiries, an account of a cure performed with electricity.

Dr. William Shippen, a pupil of John Hunter, was the first physician in America to systematize and give a full scientific course of lectures on anatomy.

He says in his letter to the trustees in September, 1765: "The institution of medical schools in this country has been a favorite object,

---

1742, Stat. Pa., ed. 1775, fol. 194; An act for the prohibiting the importation of German or other passengers in too great quantities in any one vessel, enacted 1749, Stat. Pa., ed. 1775, fol. 222; An act to encourage the establishing of an hospital for the relief of the sick poor of this province, and for the reception and cure of lunaticks, enacted 1751, Stat. Pa., ed. 1775, fol. 228; An act supplementary to the act of 1749, regarding the importation of Germans and others, enacted 1765, Stat. Pa., ed. 1775, fol. 312; An act to prevent infectious diseases being brought into this province, enacted 1774, Stat. Pa., ed. 1775, fol. 505.

occupying my attention for seven years, and it is three years since I first proposed its expediency and practicability."[1]

The fee of admission to his course was "five pistoles; and any gentlemen who incline to see the subject prepared for the lectures and learn the art of dissecting, injecting, &c., are to pay five pistoles more." The interest of these lectures was enhanced by the use of a set of large anatomical crayon-paintings and models, a then recent munificent gift of Dr. Fothergill, of London, to the Pennsylvania Hospital.

The annals of the province contain the names of many medical men who were eminent in the profession in Philadelphia prior to the Revolution and who were all zealous to advance and promote the dignity and character of medicine and medical institutions, but our space will not permit a reference to them.

PENNSYLVANIA HOSPITAL.

This excellent institution, chartered in February, 1751, had its origin in the benevolent mind of Dr. Thomas Bond, but the measure was ably seconded and its accomplishment promoted by the philanthropic Franklin and many liberal-minded citizens of the State of Pennsylvania, and it may be incidentally remarked that this institution had been from its inception, and for more than a century, identified with the progress of clinical medicine in America.

Six physicians and surgeons were appointed in 1751,[2] and arrangements made to receive patients in a temporary building. In February, 1752, the first patients entered. The new building was so far completed as to be in condition to receive patients in December, 1756.

PEST-HOUSES.

A hospital, or, as it was called, a "pest-house," was erected on Fisher's Island, afterward called Province Island. Hitherto, deserted or vacant houses on the outskirts of the city were used as temporary hospitals for the care of patients with contagious diseases.

Thomas Jefferson, in 1766, at the age of 23, went to Philadelphia to be inoculated, a cottage being rented for the purpose away from the city, near Schuylkill River.

A pest-house in Massachusetts was established as early as 1701. The necessity for hospitals of this character was caused by the frequent recurrence of the small-pox. Temporary hospitals of this character were opened in most of the colonies in which cities of any considerable size existed.

CLINICAL INSTRUCTION.

Dr. Thomas Bond, the steadfast patron and through life one of the attending physicians of the Pennsylvania Hospital, gave clinical in-

---

[1] History of the University of Pennsylvania, p. 55.

[2] Physicians and surgeons first appointed to Pennsylvania Hospital in 1751: Drs. Lloyd Zachary, Thomas Bond, Phineas Bond, Thomas Cadwallader, Samuel Preston Moore, and John Redman.—(G. B. Wood's Centennial Address, p. 12.)

struction to his class of students at the bed-side, from the opening of the institution, and in December, 1766, he submitted a nobly-conceived and well-written paper to the trustees, which has fortunately been preserved in the minutes of the journal of the institution, in which he sets forth the advantages and value of such bedside-instruction to medical students and recommends the opening of the institution, under proper regulations, to all medical students coming to Philadelphia.

MEDICAL LIBRARY OF THE PENNSYLVANIA HOSPITAL.

Out of the movement that inaugurated regular clinical instruction was developed the idea of founding the library of the Pennsylvania Hospital, which has become a great repository of medical literature and an institution of great service to the earnest student.

The plan adopted was that the fees for clinical instruction given in the hospital should be devoted, as the doctor suggested, to procuring books and preserving them for reference in the library.

The physicians of the Pennsylvania Hospital have, therefore, the credit of originating two most important measures for the advancement of medicine, namely, clinical instruction and the founding of the public medical library in the western continent.

The New York Hospital library was started in August, 1776.

EARLY PHYSICIANS IN MARYLAND.

As an evidence of the hardy and vigorous constitutions of the first *voyageurs* to the shores of Maryland, Father White, in his narration, remarks that " during the entire voyage no one was attacked with any disease;" but that, at Christmas, some having partaken immoderately of wine, which was freely distributed, thirty were seized with fever, twelve of whom died.[1]

Among the early doctors who resided in Maryland, Dr. Gerrard is mentioned as the lord of St. Clement's manor, who, it is said, in 1642, upon the ground of some claim, seized the key belonging to the chapel near the fort at St. Mary's, erected and used by the Catholics, and in which also it is probable the Anglo-Catholics or Episcopalians worshiped before the arrival of any of their ministers.[2]

This joint use of the same building for worship by separate Protestant denominations, at different hours, was at that period not unusual, and indeed it is still continued even by the Catholics and Lutherans, in some parts of Germany, to the present day.

Dr. Jacob Lumbrozo, a Jew physician in Maryland in 1649, was accused of blaspheming, but escaped a trial in consequence of the pardon accompanying the proclamation in favor of Richard, the son of the lord protector, which was issued a few days after the accusation.[3]

---

[1] Annals of Annapolis, p. 22.
[2] Davis's Day Star, p. 33.
[2] Davis's Day Star, pp. 65–66.

Dr. Luke Barber accompanied Governor Stone in his expedition in 1654 against the Puritans of Anne Arundel, for the purpose of reducing them to a submission and obedience to Lord Baltimore's government, and when they arrived at Herring's Creek the doctor and Mr. Coursey were deputed to go on before them to Providence (now Annapolis) with a proclamation addressed to the people of Anne Arundel.[1] In 1658 he was a member of the provincial court held at St. Mary's,[2] and in 1659 was one of the councilors or members of the upper house of assembly.[3]

In 1678, Edwards Husbands, a physician, was debarred, under £200 penalty, from practicing his profession[4] on account of an alleged attempt to poison the governor and council; and, for menacing and cursing the assembly, was ordered to be whipped. But he probably escaped the fine which was imposed on him and the prohibition to practice, by Lord Baltimore's dissent to the act.[5]

Drs. George Buchanan and George Walker were among the commissioners appointed in 1729, by an act entitled "An act for erecting a town on the north side of Patapsco, in Baltimore County, and for laying out into lots 60 acres of land in and about the place where one John Fleming now lives," which is the present city of Baltimore.[6]

Dr. Buchanan, a native of Scotland, purchased lands and practiced medicine in Baltimore County as early as 1723.[7] In 1745 Dr. Buchanan was appointed one of the commissioners when the towns of Baltimore and Jonestown were consolidated under the name of Baltimore Town.[8]

Dr. Walker, with his brother James, had practiced medicine in Anne Arundel for some years, but removed to Baltimore in 1715, where he died, in 1743.[9]

Dr. Dennis Claude was living in Annapolis as early as 1747, and resided in the house that was formerly the Annapolis Coffee-House.[10]

There was also a street at this time in Annapolis bearing the name of Doctor.[11] Dr. Samuel Owens was chosen delegate at the general election in 1757, and again in 1758.

Dr. William Lyon was a resident and land-owner in Baltimore in 1759.

Drs. John and Henry Stevenson were in Baltimore prior to 1763. The former conducted an extensive and prosperous trade with the parent and other European countries. The latter engaged in the practice of medicine and built a large and elegant residence near the York road.[12] In 1768 Dr. H. Stevenson converted this splendid house, which on that account was termed "Stevenson's folly," to the very laudable purpose of

---

[1] Annals of Annapolis, p. 47.
[2] Davis's Day Star, p. 66.
[3] Griffith's Sketches, Early History of Maryland, p. 18.
[4] Bacon's Laws, enacted 1678.
[5] Sketches, Early History of Mrayland, p. 29.
[6] Annals of Baltimore, p. 14.
[7] Annals of Baltimore, p. 15.
[8] Annals of Baltimore, p. 26.
[9] Ibid., p. 27.
[10] Annals of Annapolis, p. 120.
[11] Ibid., p. 121.
[12] Annals of Baltimore, p. 41.

a small-pox-infirmary, by appropriating part of it for the reception of young gentlemen, whom he inoculated successfully before the practice had become general. The practice of vaccination was promptly introduced into Maryland; and, through the zealous efforts of Dr. James Smith, thirty years later, general and free vaccination was aided by the State.[1] In 1776 Dr. Stevenson, when the colonies declared their independence, withdrew from the country. He was, however, considered a man of sterling worth.

Charles Carroll was a practitioner in Annapolis as early as 1752. In this year he had laid out and surveyed an addition to the town and the lots were advertised for sale.

Gustavus Brown, a native of Scotland, was an educated physician, and served as surgeon in the British army. In 1708 he came to Maryland. In 1711 he married a daughter of Gerard Foulke, a gentleman of large wealth. The doctor's practice was large and lucrative, often extending far into the State of Virginia. He left numerous descendants and a line of able physicians by his name, "Gustavus." He died at Port Tobacco, Md., 1765, aged 76.

Thomas Noble Stockett, a native of Maryland, was a surgeon in the Revolution. His ancestral place was near Annapolis, where he settled after the war and acquired a large professional business. He died May 16, 1802, aged 55.

Alexander Mitchell, a native of Scotland, and a well-qualified physician, practiced his profession at Bladensburg, Md., for some years, and where he died September 28, 1804, aged 36.

Gustavus Brown, a native of Maryland, was a physician of widespread professional fame, and died at his residence, "Rich Hills," near Port Tobacco, in 1804, aged 56. His medical degree was received from the University of Edinburgh. His practice for many years was very large. He was a personal friend of General Washington and was one of the physicians who were with him in his last illness.

John Nelson, a surgeon of the Revolution, died in Frederick, Md., in May, 1806. He married a Miss Washington, of Virginia.

John Archer, a native of Harford County, Md., was a patriot in the Revolution and a surgeon in the Continental Army. He was a graduate in the first medical class of the College of Philadelphia on the 21st of June, 1768, and received the degree of bachelor of medicine. He was an influential citizen and held many positions of honor in his State. An unbroken line of physicians of his descendants reside and practice with reputation in Maryland. He died in Harford County, Md., September 28, 1810, aged 69.

Charles Alexander Warfield, a patriot and a surgeon of the Revolution, died at Bushy Park, Anne Arundell County, Md., July 29, 1813. He was one of the band who burned the cargo of tea in the harbor of Annapolis just before the outbreak of the Revolution.

---
[1] Griffith's History of Maryland, p. 61.

Richard Henry Courts, a surgeon of the Revolution, practiced his profession afterward in Prince George's County, Md., up to the time of his death, in 1809.

Philip Thomas, a native of Maryland, was an eminent physician who practiced at Frederick, Md. He was president of the Medical and Chirurgical Faculty of Maryland at the time of his death, April 25, 1815. He was 68 years of age.

William Somerville practiced medicine for many years in Calvert County, Md. He removed to Baltimore, where he died, February 18 1816, aged 54.

Barton Tabbs, a native of St. Mary's County, Md., was a surgeon during the revolutionary war in the Maryland line, commanded by General Smallwood. He was a man of talent and an accomplished physician. He died in St. Mary's County, October 30, 1818, aged 61.

James Murray died at his residence in Annapolis, Md., December 17, 1819, aged 80. He had been a prominent physician in that place for nearly 60 years.

John T. Shaaf, a native of Frederick County, Md., was a practitioner of distinction at Annapolis towards the close of the last century. He then returned to Georgetown, D. C., where he practiced with success until the time of his death, April 30, 1819, at the age of 65.

John Peter Ahl, a surgeon of the Revolution, died in Baltimore, July 12, 1827, aged 78.

The following physicians were practicing in or near the town of Baltimore in 1771: Drs. Lyon, Hultz, Stenhouse, Weisenthall, Pue, Stevenson, Boyd, Craddock, Haslet, Gray, and Coulter.[1]

Dr. Weisenthall was a Lutheran and assisted in erecting a church in 1 773

In 1774 the Congress that had assembled at Philadelphia recommended the appointment of town- and county-committees throughout the colonies; and on the 12th of November, 1774, Dr. John Boyd was appointed on the committee representing Baltimore Town and County, also a member of the committee to attend the committee-meetings at Annapolis, and a member of the committee of correspondence for Baltimore.[3]

In 1774 Drs. Hultse, Weisenthall, Craddock, and Haslet were the attending physicians to the poor of Baltimore County.[4]

In 1775 James McHenry, a native of Baltimore, in company with several other gentlemen, volunteered his services to the Continental Army; he having made some progress in medicine, was appointed surgeon.[5]

In 1775 Dr. John Smith, of St. Mary's County, entered into an alliance with John Connolly, of Lancaster County, Pa., who had concocted a plan by which he could raise an army in the western parts, and there-

---

[1] Annals of Baltimore, p. 49.
[2] Annals of Baltimore, p. 36.
[3] Annals of Baltimore, p. 58.
[4] Annals of Baltimore, p. 59.
[5] Annals of Baltimore, p. 64.

by cut off all communication between the northern and southern provinces. The plan was admirably conceived and might have succeeded, were it not for the extreme vigilance of the colonists, who, having received intelligence of their designs, effected their arrest in Frederick County. Congress directed that the prisoners should be forwarded to Philadelphia. This was accordingly done, under a special guard of ten men commanded by Dr. Adam Fisher. Dr. Smith, during the journey, escaped, but was subsequently retaken, and the prisoners were safely landed in Philadelphia.

In 1776 Dr. Patrick Kennedy, after the Declaration of Independence, retired from the country, not wishing to take part in the struggle, but openly avowing before his departure that, if he could not assist, he would not oppose them. He was a man of great private virtue, and was held in high repute by the citizens.

Gustavus Brown Horner, a native of Maryland, was an eminent practitioner of medicine in Fauquier County, Virginia. He was a surgeon's mate in the war of the Revolution. After the war he settled at Warrenton, and enjoyed the patronage of a large section of the State, and was the chief surgeon for years in all important operations. He was elected to the State-legislature, was presidential elector, and held other offices to which he was chosen by an admiring community. He died July 24, 1815, aged 54.

MARYLAND SURGEONS IN THE REVOLUTION.

Drs. Jonathan Calvert, Levin Denwood, Samuel Edmonston, John L. Elbert, Ezekiel Hanie, Elisha Harrison, Samuel Y. Keene, William Kilty, Alexander Lajournade, James Mann, David Morrow, Samuel Morrow, Richard Pindell, Alexander Smith, Thomas Tillotson, Walter Warfield, and Gerard Wood, all citizens of Maryland, served as surgeons in the American revolutionary army.[1]

Clement Smith, a surgeon of the Revolution, died in Prince George's County, Md., December 10, 1831, aged 75.

Wilson Waters, a surgeon of the revolutionary war, died in Anne Arundel County, Md., February 5, 1836, aged 78.

Charles Worthington, a surgeon of the Revolution, died in Georgetown, D. C., September 10, 1836, aged 76.

John Tilden, a surgeon of the Revolution, and a minister as well as a physician, in New Town, Frederick County, Md., practiced there till the period of his death, July 21, 1838. He was 78 years of age.

---

[1] The following enactments were made in the colony of Maryland: An act for appointing coroners in each respective county, enacted 1666, Bacon's Laws of Maryland; An act establishing coroners' fees, enacted 1731, Bacon's Laws of Maryland; An act to prevent the spreading and infection of the small-pox from a vessel belonging to Amos Woodward, merchant, enacted 1731, Bacon's Laws of Maryland; An act to oblige infected ships and other vessels coming into this province to perform quarantine, enacted 1766, Stat. Md., ed. 1765–'74, fol. 158; An act to continue the foregoing act, enacted 1769, Stat. Md., 1765–74, fol. 158; An act to prevent infection from the ship Chance, enacted 1774, Stat. Md., ed. 1765–'77, fol. 393.

Henry Maynadier, a surgeon of distinction in the revolutionary war, died at Annapolis, November 11, 1849, aged 93.

Dr. Daniel Jennifer was commissioned a surgeon in the Continental Army August 26, 1776.

Ennals Martin received from the State the sum of four hundred and seventy-five pounds ten shillings and nine pence sterling as a remuneration for his meritorious services as a surgeon.

EARLY PHYSICIANS OF DELAWARE.

Henry Fiske, a native of Ireland, immigrated to America and settled to practice medicine at Lewes, Del., where he died 1748. His practice was extensive and lucrative, he often being sent for in Maryland and Pennsylvania. He had a taste for agriculture and horticulture and exercised a good influence over his section by giving practical examples of improvements, so that his place was called by his neighbors "Paradise."

Charles Ridgely, a native of Dover, Del., who, after acquiring proficiency in medicine, settled to practice in 1758, died November 25, 1785, aged 47. He was not only a good physician, but was possessed of a vast fund of knowledge in almost everything that related to the well-being of man. He was frequently sent to the legislature. Some years before the Revolution he was judge of Kent County; was a member of the committee that framed the new constitution, in 1776, for the State of Delaware.

Matthew Wilson, a native of Chester County, Pa., was a practitioner of medicine in Lewes, Del., for many years. He studied both medicine and theology, and died in 1790, aged 61. He was a man of active brain, a thorough scholar, and animated by benevolent impulses through life; was an ardent patriot, and spoke with effect against the stamp-act. He contributed many papers on medical subjects: "A therapeutic alphabet," which was never published; "The history of a malignant fever which prevailed in Sussex County, Del., in 1774," &c.

John McKinly, a native of Ireland, was a well-educated physician who settled and practiced his profession with success at Wilmington, Del. He was held in great esteem by the community; was the first governor of the State under the new constitution. He died August 31, 1796, aged 72.

Edward Miller was a native of Delaware, but in 1796 removed to the city of New York. He studied medicine with Dr. Charles Ridgely and attended lectures at the University of Pennsylvania; was a surgeon's mate in the Revolution nearly a year, in the large hospital at Baskinridge, N. J., and was surgeon for some time on a vessel employed as cruiser and bringing dispatches to France. In 1793, when yellow fever was epidemic in Philadelphia, he wrote to Dr. Rush, presenting the theory of the domestic origin. In 1796, with Dr. Elihu H. Smith and Dr. Mitchell, he projected the publication of the Medical Repository, the first medical journal in America. He was a member of nearly all the learned societies of the day and was one of the ablest medical men in the country. He died of typhus pneumonia March 17, 1812, aged 72.

George Monro, a native of New Castle, Del., was a physician of note in Wilmington during the close of the last century. He died October 11, 1819, aged 59. Towards the termination of the war he was surgeon in one of the Virginia regiments.

James Sykes, a native of Dover, Kent County, Del., practiced medicine in the same place with success during life, dying October 18, 1822, aged 61. He studied medicine with Dr. Clayton, of Bohemia Manor. He was a very popular surgeon and certainly a successful lithotomist. In 1814 he removed to New York, but in a few years returned to his native town. He was president of the State Medical Society and for nearly fifteen years was a State-senator.

George Stevenson, a surgeon of the Revolution, practiced with great repute. He was a member of the Society of Cincinnati. He died in Wilmington, Del., May 15, 1829, aged 69.

James Jones was a surgeon in the revolutionary war. He studied and practiced his profession in Duck Creek Hundred, where he died April 29, 1830, aged 74.

John Miller, a native of Dover, Del., a surgeon in the revolutionary war, died February 28, 1777, aged 25 years.

The early medical history of Delaware is much merged into that of Maryland and Pennsylvania, as the visits of the physicians of the latter States often extended into the former.

Doubtless one of the most prominent medical men of the State was James Tilton, who was born in Kent County, June 1, 1745. Having received a preliminary classical education, he entered the medical school at Philadelphia, and in 1771 obtained the degree of M. D., being a member of the first graduating class of that institution and having received the bachelor's degree in 1768.

In 1776 he entered the Army as a surgeon, but was soon promoted to the hospital-department, in which he served till the close of the war. In 1785 he was made commissioner of loans and at the breaking-out of the war of 1812 was appointed physician and Surgeon-General of the Army. He was also a member of the Congress sitting at Philadelphia. He died near Wilmington, May 14, 1822. Seven years previous (when at the age of 70) he had his leg amputated on account of disease of the knee-joint.

Reuben Gilder and Henry Latimer, of this State, served as surgeons in the Continental Army and John B. Cutting as apothecary. The last-named died February 3, 1831, in the District of Columbia.

Joshua Clayton, a native of Delaware, died of yellow fever in 1799 at an advanced age. He was an intelligent physician and a most exemplary citizen. During the revolutionary war, when Peruvian bark was scarce, he was led to use a combination of the bark of the poplar (*Lirodendron*) and the dogwood (*Cornus florida*) as a substitute, and with good results, he thought. He was president of the State for many years, and after the war, and the adoption of the Constitution, was chosen governor. He was also United States Senator.

GEORGIA SURGEONS IN THE REVOLUTION.

Jacob V. Egbert, James Houston, James B. Sharpe, Benjamin Tetard, and John G. Wright, physicians of Georgia, served as surgeons in the Continental Army.

SURGEONS NOT LOCATED.

John Applewhaite; John Wingate, who died in Kennebec County, Maine, July 25, 1819; Felix Texier; John Roberts, who died in Franklin County, Kentucky, April 21, 1821; Elisha Skinner, who died in Penobscot County, Maine, November, 1827; John Knight; Corbin Griffin, who was surgeon of the hospital at Yorktown, and Ezra Green served as surgeons to the American Army during the revolutionary war, but of what States they were citizens previous to entering the military service is not easy to ascertain.

SURGEONS AT BUNKER HILL.

The following-named physicians were attached to the American forces and rendered professional assistance to the patriots at the battle of Bunker Hill: Isaac Foster, John Hart, Walter Hastings, David Jones, David Townsend, Obadiah Williams, and Lieut. Col. James Bricket. The last-mentioned, although an officer of the line, gave surgical aid to the wounded in that memorable battle.[1]

Able physicians were located throughout the colonies not specially mentioned. They possessed, however, no large centers of population or leading educational institutions around which to cluster and gain permanent professional recognition. Their works, when noticed, have gone to swell the reputation of the profession in general in America.

ENDEMICS AND EPIDEMICS.

The following list of diseases comprises the names of those that most frequently and severely afflicted the early settlers in America and which the colonial physician was called upon to treat. The mortality attending some of these diseases, when the epidemic proved to be wide-spread, was very great, and would be alarming at the present. That the diseases here enumerated, or most of them, have prevailed, either in an endemic or in an epidemic[2] form, at different times and places, cannot be doubted;

---

[1] In Delaware, in 1726, a law entitled "An act to prevent infected vessels coming into this Government," and which was revised in 1797, was enacted, and is the only one that I can discover appertaining to either hygiene or medicine passed during the period of the colonial Government.—Revised Stat. Delaware, vol. 1, fol. 98.

[2] The term epidemic is, I apprehend, often applied unadvisedly and where the facts when examined do not justify its use. This is particularly true of the past, but the profession has adopted no definite rule for its application. What degree of prevalence

but I do not wish to be understood as asserting that I have included all, and none but those that are entitled to be mentioned.

I have omitted many localities where particular diseases were said to be prevailing as an epidemic, because it appeared to me the facts did not justify the application of the term. I must ask, therefore, that the lists be taken as nearly approximating the data collected.

It would occupy unnecessary space to give all the authorities in every instance from which the facts have been collated.[1] I have adopted the simplest possible form, by grouping the facts, by taking the name of the disease, and then giving the name of each locality and the year of its appearance with severity and re-appearance at that place. Although the list is incomplete, it will possess interest.[2]

---

of a disease should entitle it to be so denominated? New Orleans, a city that, perhaps, has been constrained to declare the existence of epidemics prevailing within its boundaries oftener than other within the United States, has acted upon the idea that where any particular disease caused more deaths than occurred from all other causes and diseases, then the unusual and chief-prevailing disease has been declared to be epidemic. It is needless to say that in the use of the term a larger latitude is given than statistical accuracy demands.

[1] The following are some of the works consulted: Webster on Epidemics, Smith on Typhus, Morris Scarlet Fever, Tennent's Epistle, Thacher's History of Medicine, Gallup on Epidemic Diseases of Vermont, Ramsey's State of Medicine in the Eighteenth Century, and numerous State- and local histories.

[2] *Small-pox:* New England, 1618, 1622, 1638, 1721, 1730, 1752; New York, 1721, 1731, 1752; Salem, Mass., 1633, 1711, 1792; New Jersey, 1730, 1752, 1764; Charleston, S. C., 1699, 1700, 1717, 1732, 1738, 1760; Philadelphia, 1730, 1731, 1732, 1736, 1756; Williamsburg, Va., 1748, 1765; Boston, 1631, 1633, 1639, 1645, 1647, 1649, 1666, 1677, 1678, 1689, 1701, 1702, 1721, 1730, 1752, 1764, 1776, 1792; Pennsylvania, 1661, 1663, 1732, 1757; Virginia, 1748, 1752, 1764; Lancaster, Pa., 1757; Maryland, 1730, 1757, 1764; Annapolis, Md., 1757.

Nervous fever: Wethersfield, Conn., 1793; Albany, N. Y., 1746.

Yellow fever: New London, Conn., 1798; Wilmington, Del., 1798; Boston, Mass., 1691, 1693, 1796, 1798; Holliston, Mass., 1741; Nantucket, Mass., 1763; New Design, Md., 1797; Portsmouth, N. H., 1798; Albany, N. Y., 1746; New York, N. Y., 1668, 1702, 1732, 1741, 1743, 1791, 1795, 1798, 1799; Chester, Pa., 1798; Philadelphia, Pa., 1699, 1741, 1762, 1793, 1797, 1798, 1799; Providence, R. I., 1795, 1797; Charleston, S. C., 1699, 1700, 1703, 1728, 1732, 1739, 1745, 1748, 1749, 1753, 1755, 1758, 1792, 1794, 1795, 1796, 1797, 1799, 1800; New Orleans, La., 1769, 1791, 1793, 1794, 1795, 1797, 1799, 1800; Mobile, Ala., 1705, 1766; Pensacola, Fla., 1764.

Plague, (probably yellow fever:) New Haven, 1794; Philadelphia, 1740, 1762, 1778, 1780, 1794, 1797, 1798; New York, 1702, 1743, 1745, 1794, 1795, 1796, 1798; Baltimore, 1783, 1794, 1797; Mill River, Conn., 1795; Nantucket, 1763; Martha's Vineyard, 1763; Virginia, 1660, 1695, 1737, 1740; Mohegan Indians, 1745, 1746; Marcus Hook, Wilmington, (Del.,) New Castle, (Del.,) Duck Creek, Bridgeton, (N. J.,) Woodbury, (N. J.,) 1798; Norfolk, Conn., 1797, 1798; Boston, 1693, 1698, 1795, 1798; Portsmouth, New London, 1798; Wilmington, N. C., 1796; Charleston, 1728, 1732, 1740, 1746, 1796, 1797; Newburyport, Mass., 1796; Providence, 1797; Connecticut, 1662, 1683.

Scarlatina: Connecticut, 1751, 1793, 1794; Vermont, 1787, 1793, 1796, 1797; Windsor, Bethel, Stockbridge, Barnard, Royalton, Woodstock, Randolph, 1795; Philadelphia, 1746, 1764, 1783, 1789, 1793, 1794; Kingston, Mass., 1735; Boston, 1702, 1735, 1795; Ulster, 1785; New England, 1787; New Haven, 1793, 1794; New York, 1792, 1793, 1794; Salem, Mass., 1783; Charlestown, 1784; North Fairfield, 1793; Massachusetts, 1793, 1796; Hart-

REASONS FOR STUDYING ABROAD.

If the supply of really competent teachers was limited under the conditions and wants of our new country, the student-class which could have been drawn together at any one of the colonial capitals was also small. The rivalries natural between the different communities prevented concert of action and a concentration of resources.

The lines of travel between the States were then undeveloped, and it was almost as easy for a medical student to cross the Atlantic and attend the University of Padua or Leyden as to have attended a school, if one had existed, in a remote province in America.

During the opening years of the eighteenth century the attractions of those continental seats of learning were unsurpassed and their authority in science absolute. To Leyden in particular, that Athens of the

ford, 1794; New Hampshire, Me., 1796; Bethlehem, Conn., 1792, 1793, 1794; Litchfield, 1793; New Jersey, Redbrook, 1789.

Dysentery: North America, 1752, 1758; Woodbury, Conn., 1749; Hartford, Conn., 1751; New Haven, Conn., 1751, 1773, 1795; Middletown, Conn., 1775; Dutchess County, N. Y., 1795; New York, 1709, 1739, 1776; Danbury, 1775; Mt. Independence, 1776; Georgetown, Md., 1793; Derby, 1794; Salem, Mass., 1773; Coventry, Conn., 1793; Stamford, Conn., 1745; Connecticut, 1749; Waterbury, Conn., 1749; Cornwall, Conn., 1749; Virginia, 1635; Hanover, Vt., 1798; Farmington, Vt., 1798; Bennington, Vt., 1782, 1788; Vermont, 1776; Rutland, 1796; Landgate, Vt., 1798; Bethlehem, Conn., 1798; Portland, 1797; Sheffield, 1795; Wilmington, 1795.

Typhus: Hartford, North Haven, East Haven, New Haven, (Conn.,) 1760; Bethlehem; Conn., 1760, 1797; Windsor, Royalton, Bethel, Randolph, Pomfret, Birmingham, Stockbridge, Arlington, (Vt.,) Norwich, (Conn.,) 1798; Woodstock, Vt., 1799; Royalton, 1798; Cornish, N. H., 1798; Dover, N. H., 1697; Dutchess County, N. Y., 1795; Byberry, Moreland, (Pa.,) 1793.

Malignant fever: New York, 1745, 1787; Fredericktown, Md., 1788; Portland, 1797; New York, 1668.

Angina: Kingston, N. H., 1733, 1734, 1735; Boston, 1735, 1769; Northampton. Mass., 1787; New England, 1737, 1742, 1787; Connecticut, 1751; Long Island, 1755; Massachusetts, 1736.

Measles: Massachusetts, 1713, 1739, 1769, 1773; Charleston, S. C., 1747, 1759, 1772, 1775; Philadelphia, 1771, 1773, 1788, 1796; Connecticut, 1740; New York, 1788, 1795; Vermont, 1788.

Sore throat: Long Island, N. Y., 1769; Vermont, 1773, 1783; Eastern States, 1786; 1787; Kingston, (N. H.,) Exeter, (N. H.,) Boston, Chester, 1735; America, 1773; Philadelphia, 1763.

Influenza: New York, 1789; Philadelphia, 1760, 1761, 1789; Bethlehem, Conn., 1760; Massachusetts, 1697, 1761, 1781, 1789; Vermont, 1789, 1790, 1798; Boston, 1734, 1737; Fairfield, 1697; Charlestown, 1778.

Catarrh: Massachusetts, 1747, 1756, 1772; Vermont, 1781, 1790; New York, 1789; Philadelphia, 1719, 1773, 1790, 1794; Hartford, 1739, 1790; Boston, 1789; New England, 1655, 1658; Albany, 1790.

Croup: Middletown, Conn., 1775; Bethlehem, Conn., 1792; Connecticut, 1659.

Pleurisy: New York, 1749; Shaftsbury, Vt., 1786; Waterbury, Conn., 1712; Hartford, Conn., 1719; Philadelphia, 1794.

Fever: Bethlehem, Conn., 1750; Cape Cod, Mass., 1772; Philadelphia, 1793; Charleston, S. C., 1739; Holliston, Conn., 1742; Boston, 1745; New York, 1619, 1732; America, 1638; Connecticut, 1647; Wood Creek, N. Y., 1709; Charleston, 1761.

Canker-rash: Vermont, 1787, 1796.

John Tennent, in a letter to Dr. Richard Mead, of London, in 1738, mentions that in

West, and to the eloquent Booerhaave and his able *confrères*, were turned the thoughts of those who aspired to enter the profession, and by travel to obtain more professional knowledge than was to be acquired at home.

After the death of Booerhaave, Edinburgh, with Cullen as its great light, became the favorite resort of American students. The standard of preparatory training then required was much higher than at present, especially in the languages, for most of the text-books were written in Latin and Greek, and all lectures were delivered in Latin prior to 1746, when Cullen, who dared to innovate the established custom, lectured in English.

Graduates were required to present, publish, and defend a thesis in one of the learned languages. Such high requirements virtually closed the doors of the profession, except to the well-educated.

When we consider that the Edinburgh School of Medicine, an institution with which Cullen united in 1756, organized about 1700 and not fully established until about 1725, was the first under the British government to achieve eminent success, it is not surprising that her distant colonies were backward in founding medical colleges.

The Wind-mill Street School of Anatomy was founded by the Hunters in 1770. Prior to this period dissection was seldom required or practiced by the students, they being merely present at the demonstrations of the professor in the lecture-room, where he often taught from models and drawings, and without a fresh subject before him.

FOUNDING OF MEDICAL SCHOOLS AT HOME.

From this cursory view of the surroundings of medical men at home and abroad, the establishment of two medical schools in America appears highly creditable to our people, who had an ardent craving for knowledge, as well as to the intelligence and enterprise of the professional men of that period.

MEDICAL COLLEGE OF PHILADELPHIA.

Drs. Shippen and Morgan, already mentioned, both natives of that city and graduates of Edinburgh, had, while studying their profession abroad, concerted a plan for establishing a regular medical school, at an early day, in their own country.

Virginia, " From the first of June to August continued periodical fevers and intermittents are epidemical, and then agues precede the latter till October, when pleurisies and peripneumonies begin to be common, and continue till May or June, tho' seldom epidemic."—(John Tennent's epistle to Dr. R. Mead, p. 12.)

Bilious fever: Philadelphia, 1778, 1780.

The diseases most prevalent in New England were the following: Alvine fluxes, Saint Anthony's fire, asthma, atrophy, catarrh, colic; inflammatory, slow, nervous, and mixed fevers; pulmonary consumption, quinzy, rheumatism.—(Winterbotham's America, vol. 2, p. 3.)

Their plan when presented at home was received with favor, and in 1765 the medical department of the College of Philadelphia (a well-established literary institution, founded in 1749) was organized under two professorships, which comprised all the branches, the one in the name of "theory and practice of physic," held by Dr. Morgan; the other in "anatomy and surgery," filled by Dr. Shippen.[1]

The Medical College of Philadelphia was fully organized in May, 1765, although it may be said to have had an earlier beginning, as a systematic course of lectures on anatomy had been delivered to respectable classes from the year 1762.

The College of New York was founded in 1767 and fully organized in 1768. Dr. Samuel Clossy, however, had commenced a private course of anatomical lectures in 1764.

While high honor is due to the New England colonies for their early, generous, persistent, and judicious efforts in the cause of general education and literature, they accomplished less for medical science prior to the Revolution, and, indeed, in the last century, than might have been expected.

The first course of lectures of Dr. Shippen, on anatomy, already alluded to, was given to twelve students, in a room in the rear of his own office, and continued every year to increased classes, from 1762 until 1765, when the college opened, after which he taught, in addition to anatomy, surgery and obstetrics. It was about this period that a mob attacked his anatomical rooms, on account of his leadership in teaching anatomy and persisting in the dissection of the human body for such purposes, in the face of the prejudices of the age.

His subjects at this time were supplied from the few criminals and suicides, which latter had been granted by public and governmental authority.

The "doctors' mob" in 1788 marked the last serious resistance of the populace to the teaching of practical anatomy in America, although

---

[1] It is difficult to ascertain the precise period of the formation and establishment of the great universities of Europe, or at least of the older ones among them. But about the beginning of the twelfth century a number of them acquired importance and influence. Then it was that the custom of conferring degrees and academic honors was established and became general. The degree of bachelor was the first conferred; then master; then doctor; and the same gradation is still retained. The first degree of doctor was, I believe, conferred by the University of Bologna, about A. D. 1130. Iruerius, the "Lucerna juris," who died at Bologna in 1150, is said to have drawn up the first formula for the degree "*Juris utriusque doctor*," which was conferred upon Bulgarus. The University of Paris adopted the degree in 1145. The first recipients of the degree of "*Sacræ theologiæ doctor*" were Peter Lombard, who died in 1164, and Gilbert de la Potrée, the two leading divines of their day.

Sir Henry Spelman, a learned antiquary, born in 1561, thinks the title "doctor" was not used till after the publication of Lombard's Sentences, about 1140, and affirms that "such as explained that work to their scholars first received the appellation of doctors."

Others claim that Bede, surnamed "the venerable," who died in 735, aged 63, was the first doctor of Cambridge, and that John Beverly, a learned bishop, who founded

enactments long remained unrepealed, in the statutes of some of the States, which greatly embarrassed the colleges in procuring material for the dissecting-room, but they have been either repealed or become obsolete.

This desultory narration of the attempts at instruction in anatomy and surgery covers the fifteen years beginning with 1750 and brings us to the decade immediately preceding the Revolution. The times were then (1765) ripe for a higher, a better-organized, and a more efficient home professional education. Men eminently fitted for the undertaking were at hand and the era of systematic public teaching in medicine opened in Philadelphia, then the principal commercial city of the North American provinces.

A third chair was filled, in 1768, by the election of Dr. Adam Kuhn as professor of materia medica and botany. Dr. Thos. Bond, a native

---

a college at Oxford and died in 721, was the first at that university; but Spelman will not allow that "doctor" was the name of any title or degree in England prior to the reign of King John, about 1207.

The title, from its earliest use, was held in great estimation by different faculties, as is evidenced by the doctors contending with knights for precedence; which disputes were in many instances terminated by advancing the doctors to the dignity of knighthood.

The degree of "doctor" was a certificate that the person receiving it was competent to teach the branch for which it was conferred. The faculties recognized, in which the degree was given, were theology, philosophy, law, medicine, and the arts, (or polite literature.) Philosophy and the arts could not in any country, and least of all in England, become professions with a numerous following. The individual who had pursued his studies so far as to receive the degree of doctor in them either went further, and devoted himself to theology, law, or medicine, or else became attached to the universities, and never became so familiar with the people as to fix upon his class the popular appellation of "doctor." The title was well known and frequent in the profession of law, but only of the civil or Roman law, prevalent in Southern Europe. The common law of England was never taught in the English universities until a quite recent date, not 150 years ago; and the degree of doctor of the common law never existed. The English were the only people of modern times who produced a system of law, original and entire in itself and wholly differing from the common civil law which obtains elsewhere throughout Christendom. Even in the earliest times, the English were particularly jealous to guard against any inroads on their system of common law by the Roman or civil lawyers, and hence their schools of jurisprudence were not established at any of the academic colleges, but at the Inns of Court, near Westminster Hall, where, in their peculiar way and in antagonism to the schools of civil law, they gave, instead of the degrees of bachelor and doctor, the rank of barrister and sergeant, titles now well known in England in the higher walks of the profession.

Hence the title of doctor could never have been popularly applied to the lawyers. To the faculties, therefore, of divinity and medicine must its common use necessarily have been confined. But the doctorate of the clergyman, though it yet exists and is in frequent use, was and is sunk in his character of priest or bishop, and other reverential appellations, derived from their spiritual functions, as father, friar, (brother,) &c., or indicative of their office in the church, as bishop, curate, abbot, prior, pastor, &c.; and the title of doctor remained in the almost exclusive possession of the medical fraternity, and conveyed the idea that they were appointed by authority to give directions for the management of the sick and the preparation and administration of medicines.

of Maryland, already mentioned, had been in 1768 elected professor of clinical medicine.

Dr. Benjamin Rush, in 1769, was elected professor of chemistry.

By these five gentlemen medical teaching was conducted until the city of Philadelphia was occupied by the British army, in 1777. In some of the sessions, the classes numbered above thirty students.

Three of the professors accepted places in the Continental Army and Navy—Shippen, Morgan, and Rush. The number of graduates, during the first decade of the Philadelphia school, was but twenty-eight, all of whom received the bachelor's degree. Four of those, however, again presented themselves in 1771, and, having published a thesis in Latin and having passed an examination in public in the same language, obtained the degree of doctor of medicine.

It can be readily understood that, when there was no standard of preparatory education demanded of a student before commencing the study, nor any obligation to give evidence of due knowledge and professional qualifications to allow them the privilege to practice, preliminary education would certainly become lowered in the profession.

Many went directly from their preceptor's office and commenced their professional career, without attending lectures or obtaining even a license from any department of the Government. The necessities of a new country and the limited pecuniary means of students pleaded in their favor with the community and induced them generally to commence the practice of their profession after attending one course of lectures or receiving the " bachelor's degree."

The cares of a home and of a practice already acquired in a rural and sparsely-settled country prevented many, every way worthy of the honor, from returning to the college to receive the degree of doctor of medicine. Two of the graduates of the class of 1768-'71—Jonathan Potts and James Tilton—became distinguished physicians and held important and responsible positions in the medical department of the revolutionary Army. The bachelors, in graduating, participated in the public exercises, which, for the most part, were in Latin.

Since 1812 the degree of doctor of medicine is the only one granted in any of our American medical colleges.

Dr. Morgan, in his address at the commencement of the college in 1765, said:

"Perhaps this medical institution, the first of its kind in America, though small in its beginning, may receive a constant accession of strength and annually exert new vigor.

"It may collect a number of young persons of more than ordinary abilities, and so improve their knowledge as to spread its reputation to different parts.

"By sending these abroad, duly qualified, or by exciting an emulation among men of parts and literature, it may give birth to other useful institutions of a similar nature or occasional rise by its example to numerous societies of different kinds, calculated to spread the light of knowledge through the whole American continent, wherever inhabited."[1]

A part of this prediction soon received its verification.

EARLY PHYSICIANS IN NEW HAMPSHIRE.

Nathaniel Rogers, a native of Portsmouth, N. H., studied medicine and practiced in his native place. He was a graduate of Harvard College and studied with Dr. Bailey, of Ipswich. His practice was very large until the time of his death, which took place in 1745, at the age of 45.

Nathaniel Sargent, a native of New England, practiced medicine in Portland, N. H. He studied medicine with Dr. Packer and commenced to practice in Hampton, but on the death of Dr. Pierce he removed to Portland, where he died, in June, 1762.

Dr. Ezra Carter, a native of the State, died at Concord, where he had practiced his profession, September 17, 1794, aged 48. He studied with Dr. Ordway, of Salisbury, Mass.

Dr. William Coggswell, of N. H., was a surgeon in the Revolution. He remained in charge of the hospital at West Point until 1785, when it was closed.

Petetiah Warren, a surgeon of the Revolution settled to practice at Berwick, Me. He was from New Hampshire, and served as surgeon's mate in the Second New Hampshire Regiment, in 1776. In 1785 he sailed from Salem, Mass., for the coast of Africa, but never returned.

Clement Jackson practiced medicine with distinction at Portsmouth, N. H., through a long life. He died in 1788, aged 82. His son, Hall Jackson, also studied medicine and rose to eminence in the profession. He died in 1797.

William Parker was a surgeon in the Revolution; after the war he settled at Exeter, N. H., where he acquired a leading business, which he retained to the time of his death, which occurred September 15, 1798, from an attack of yellow fever.

Josiah Bartlett was a good physician and an ardent patriot in the Revolution. Having completed his professional studies he commenced to practice in Kingston, N. H., at the age of 21. He enjoyed a large practice, was exceedingly popular as a citizen, was a member of the Colonial Congress, and was a signer of the Declaration of Independence. He was governor of the State, president of the State Medical Society, and justice of the supreme court. He was able and faithful in every position. He died of paralysis, May 19, 1795, aged 65.

Joshua Brackett, a native of New Hampshire, was a physician of excellent ability; resided and practiced in Portsmouth, N. H., where he died, July 17, 1802, aged 69. He was a graduate of Harvard College in 1752. His medical studies were prosecuted under Dr. Clement Jackson. He was an honorary member of the Massachusetts Medical So-

---

[1] Discourse upon the Institution of Middle Schools in America, p. 58.

ciety. The honorary degree of M. D. was conferred upon him by his *alma mater* in 1793. He succeeded Dr. Bartlett in the presidency of the New Hampshire Medical Society. He gave 143 volumes of valuable books to the State Medical Society to form a library. His wife subsequently gave a donation of $1,500 towards the same purpose.

Ezra Green was a surgeon of the Revolution, who after the war settled and practiced his profession at Dover, N. H., with success until near the end of his life. He died in the year 1847, at the age of 101 years and 28 days. He was a graduate of Harvard in 1765. He was for a time surgeon on board the Ranger, commanded by Paul Jones.

Dr. Samuel Curtis, of Amherst, N. H., was a surgeon on board the frigate Hancock, commanded by Capt. John Manly. He also served on other vessels in the same capacity during the Revolution. He died March 27, 1822, aged 74.

MEDICAL COLLEGE OF NEW YORK.

In New York, in 1768, the second medical college in the New World was fully organized as a department of King's (now Columbia) College, which had been founded in 1754. Like the Philadelphia school, it came into being in consequence of the efforts of physicians who had already been engaged in private instruction, Dr. Clossy having commenced a course of lectures on anatomy in 1763.

Drs. Middleton and Clossy were elected to the chairs of theory of physic and anatomy; the other members of the faculty were Drs. Samuel Bard, professor of the practice of physic; James Smith, of chemistry and materia medica; John V. B. Tennant, of midwifery, and John Jones, of surgery.

The four professors last named were Americans and had completed their education in European universities. Seldom has a school opened with so numerous and competent a corps of teachers. Of the seven branches usually taught at the present day, this institution had six. Physiology, the seventh branch, was not then sufficiently matured to justify a separate chair, and clinical medicine was not included for the reason that there was at that time no general hospital in the city of New York.

The corner-stone of the New York Hospital was laid July 27, 1773, and the building was unfortunately destroyed by fire just as it reached completion, in 1775, and before it had been occupied.

The curriculum of study in these schools was modeled upon that of the University of Edinburgh, from which nearly all the professors had graduated. The standard of requirements governing the examination of candidates for degrees was high and about the same in each.

The medical department of Harvard University, Massachusetts, was organized and lectures began in 1782.

The organization of the medical department of Dartmouth College, N. H., was completed in 1797.

These four were the chief medical schools organized in America up to the close of the eighteenth century. At the present time there are hundreds of all grades.

RULES OF ADMISSION AND EXAMINATION.

It will suffice to indicate the most important rules adopted on this point. First, such students as have not taken a degree in arts must give evidence of a competent knowledge of Latin and of certain branches of natural philosophy. Secondly, three years after matriculation, an examination for the bachelor's degree will be allowed to students who have taken one complete course of lectures. Thirdly, one year after obtaining the primary degree the student will be admitted to examination for the doctorate, if he shall be 22 years of age, shall have attended two full courses of lectures, and have published and publicly defended a treatise upon some medical subject. Fourthly, the mode of examination shall follow that of the most celebrated universities of Europe.

DATE OF FIRST DEGREES.

The first bachelor's degree conferred in America was granted in Philadelphia in 1768 and in New York in 1769. The first degree of doctor in medicine was conferred in New York in 1770 and in Philadelphia in 1771. The first medical degree conferred by the University of Edinburgh was in 1705.

ANNUAL SESSIONS.

The regular course of lectures generally began in September and closed in May or June. Dr. Shippen's course in anatomy embraced sixty lectures. The practice of delivering introductory lectures was in vogue from the first, and two or more of them pronounced at the opening of these schools were printed and are still in existence.

Copies of the published thesis of the first graduates are also extant.[1]

The cost to a student of taking a bachelor's degree was not far from $60 of the money of the present day.

PROGRESS OF MEDICAL EDUCATION.

To those who have noted the conditions and events in the colonies, narrated in the preceding pages, affecting the medical profession, it will be evident that the means and facilities available to young men preparing to enter the profession, before the Revolution, were so meager that they can scarcely be conceived by either the practitioner or student of the present day. As a general fact, in early times the young man was apprenticed to his preceptor for from three to seven years, the student,

---

[1] See Catalogue of Library of the Surgeon-General's Office.

too, in most cases, beginning professional studies at the early age of from 14 to 18. It will naturally be inferred from this that many of the students were less qualified by preparatory education for commencing professional studies than was desirable. Indeed, it was not an unusual thing that the student, in addition to his medical reading, was at the same time receiving instruction in the languages, either at an academy, from his medical preceptor, or some neighboring clergyman. This was particularly true in rural districts, in which the higher schools or academies were scarce. The usages of European countries were, as a matter of course, brought over by the early settlers and made the basis of social customs, professional regulations, and local laws. In the Old World, it had been the practice for centuries for the medical student to be apprenticed for a term of about seven years to his preceptor.[1] This custom, although gradually yielding, lingered longest in the rural districts and smaller towns, whence came most of our early settlers.

The system of apprenticeship in the profession of medicine was still in vogue in America up to the period of the independence of the colonies and in some of the States to a late period. Many young men of good preparatory education, with ample pecuniary means to pursue their professional studies, were indentured for terms of years. This indentureship was a sort of servitude on the part of the young man, and contracted that he should be taught the science and art of medicine, and that he should give all his time and energy to the study and to whatever other business-interests his preceptor might require of him. With great propriety this always included the compounding of prescriptions and the prepar-

---

[1] The system or practice of apprenticing youths for a term of years, usually seven, originated at a period when the genteel professions, trades, and most other pursuits were almost exclusively carried on by corporate institutions. The custom of conducting professions and business through guilds and corporations became so general in the fifteenth century as almost to paralyze individual energies. They were, in England, finally restricted in their powers during the reign of Elizabeth. The guilds, of a semi-military character, probably had their origin in the free cities of Italy, where the trades-people had to defend themselves against the rapacity of the lords. These associations adopted and fostered democratic and independent principles of government in their societies. In progress of time, in different countries, they became the strong arm for protecting the citizens' rights and liberties. Countries where the guilds of various kinds flourished most took the lead in reforms that have ameliorated the condition of the mass of the people. By the close of the twelfth century guilds were common throughout Europe, particularly in Italy, Germany, and Great Britain; and although they were, at one period in the progress of civilization, of great importance to the people, they in time became intolerable aristocracies and oppressive to individual industry and enterprise, so that their restriction became a necessity. The lawyer, as well as the physician, a century or two back, in receiving a young man as a student, had him indentured; and, although seven years was the usual time, the period was a matter to be determined by the contracting parties. The barrister frequently studied sixteen years, after which he might take the degree of sergeant—"*servitudos ad legem.*" In our country, instances occurred of clergymen taking apprentices to teach them theology and prepare them regularly for the universities of particular denominations.

ation of medicines. Formerly medicines were furnished to physicians and drug-stores in their crude form, as imported. To pulverize bark and roots, to make and spread plasters, to make tinctures, ointments, extracts, and blue-mass, &c., was the arduous labor of days. The students were commonly intrusted with bleeding, cupping, pulling teeth, dressing minor wounds, attending to night-calls in the office, and occasionally visiting patients with their preceptor.

The sparseness of population in the rural districts, the limited pecuniary means of many students, and their inability to board at home or to find boarding-places in the vicinity of the doctor's office necessitated the student to become an inmate of his preceptor's family. Relations of this character naturally served to identify intimately the student's life with all that affected the reputation and success of his preceptor and which dignified all duties and labors.

Prof. Dunglison, in the Medical Student, pages 59, 60, in speaking of the student-life in the office of a preceptor in England, says: "He instructs him, moreover, to bleed, glyster, draw teeth, &c.; and not many years ago it was the practice in some of the country-places of England, and perhaps still is, to require that the medical pupil should attend to the horse, if his employer kept one, see that it was regularly groomed, fed, and watered, and bring it saddled to the door on all sudden emergencies! What an employment for the future member of a liberal and learned profession! and what a waste of time in a pupilage, thus unnecessarily protracted."

What is here given as a picture of the student's life in Great Britain may be taken as applicable to the profession at an early period in the colonies. Dr. John Bard, in 1732, at the age of between 14 and 15 years, according to the custom of the times, was bound apprentice for seven years to Mr. Kearsley, one of the leading surgeons of Philadelphia, but a man of unhappy temper. "He treated his pupils with great rigor and subjected them to the most menial employments, to which Dr. Bard has been heard to say he would never have submitted but from the apprehension of giving pain to his excellent mother, who was then a widow with seven children and a very moderate income, and from the encouragement he received from the kindness of her particular friend, Mrs. Kearsley, of whom he always spoke in terms of the warmest gratitude, affection, and respect." (Thacher's Medical Biography, p. 97.) Dr. Benjamin Rush, in 1760, after acquiring a classical education, was apprenticed at the age of 15 to Dr. John Redman for six years. He was in daily attendance upon the shop of his preceptor, and it was during this time that he wrote the only account we have of the yellow fever in Philadelphia of 1762. Dr. James Lloyd, of Boston, at the age of 17, in 1745 commenced his medical studies, which continued for nearly five years, under Dr. Clark, of Boston. Dr. Daniel Drake, in 1800, "commenced his pupilage with Dr. Goforth in his sixteenth year. During the next three years his chief occupation was the study of medicine, the running of errands, the compounding of drugs, and all such employments as befall a country doctor's boy, student, young man, or whatever else bluntness or courtesy might call him." (Mansfield's Life of Drake, p. 54.) It would be quite easy to add the names of other distinguished American physicians who were apprenticed to their medical preceptor.

From the constant struggle that was incumbent on all classes of society to provide the necessary means of life, high literary culture was exceptional or had to be in a measure overlooked, even by the medical profession. There were but a few towns up to the period of the Revolution where the population was great enough to bring together a sufficient number of physicians to enable them to form a society either for professional discussion and advancement or for social intercourse.

The aggregate population of the colonies in 1776 was perhaps not much in excess of 3,000,000. The first census taken by authority of Congress was in 1790, when the number of inhabitants was found to be 3,928,326. In 1800 the returns gave 5,319,762. It is estimated that there was about one physician for every 800 of the population in towns and one for about every ten or twelve hundred throughout the rural districts.[1]

There were probably not 3,500 physicians all told in the United States when the colonies declared themselves independent of Great Britain.

[1] *Table of the towns of over 5,000 population in the different States in 1790 and 1800, made up from the United States census-reports.*

Towns.	Population 1790.	Population 1800.	Towns.	Population 1790.	Population 1800.
Portsmouth, N. H		5,339	*Ballstown, Albany County, N. Y.	7,333	
Boston, Mass	18,038	24,937	*Frederickstown, Dutchess County, N. Y	5,932	
*Gloucester, Essex County, Mass	5,317	5,331	*Fishkill, Dutchess County, N. Y.	5,941	6,168
*Marblehead, Mass	5,661	5,211	*Rennselaerwicktown, Albany County, N. Y	8,318	5,541
*Newburyport, Mass		5,946			
*Salem, Mass	7,921	9,457	Schenectady City, Albany County, N. Y		5,389
Providence, R. I	6,380	7,614	*Stephentown, Albany County, N. Y	6,795	
*Newport, R. I	6,716	6,539			
*Hartford, Conn		5,347	*Stephentown, Rennselaer County, N. Y		5,948
*Middleton, Conn		5,001			
*New London, Conn		5,150	*Washington, Dutchess County, N. Y	5,189	
*Norwalk, Conn		5,196	*Watervliet, Albany County, N.Y.	7,419	
*Stonington, Conn		5,537	Philadelphia, Pa	45,250	70,287
Albany, N. Y		5,289	Baltimore, Md	13,503	26,114
New York, N. Y	33,131	60,489	Richmond, Va		5,737
*Canaan Town, Columbia County, N. Y	6,692		*Charleston, S. C	16,359	20,563
*Connasacharrie, Montgomery County, N. Y	6,156		*Savannah, Ga		5,166
*Cambridge, Washington County, N. Y		6,187	*Christiana, Del		6,328
*Clinton, Dutchess County, N. Y		5,203			

The United States census-returns do not afford the data for an exact statement of the populations of the towns of the different colonies. Some of the towns include villages and townships or even a larger civil division. This is offered only as an approximate list; a more careful study would probably add to it Lancaster, Pa.; and a few other places ought perhaps to be included. Places marked with an asterisk (*) are supposed to comprehend the inhabitants of the township as well as corporate borough.

It is further probable that there were not much, if any, over 350 who had received a medical degree.

If we make the general average of one physician for every 800 of the population, it would give us 4,970 physicians in 1790, and in 1800 the same rate of physicians to total population would give 6,649 physicians for the United States; or, if we adopt the ratio of physicians to total population furnished by the late census, which is one physician to every 618 persons, there would have been, in 1790, 6,324 physicians, and, in 1800, 8,608. I am satisfied, however, that even the first estimate is too high for the period of our history antedating the Revolution. There were but a few towns then with a population of over 5,000, and consequently the opportunity for professional intercourse, even if the medical practitioners were inclined, was not great. In the rural districts, the pioneer was constantly battling to subdue the forest and protect himself against the elements. He had but little time to indulge in literary pursuits or to enjoy such acquirements in others. There always has been, and always must be, a relation between the qualifications of the medical practitioner of a country and the degree of culture and the necessities for individual labor on the part of the mass of the people.

It is probable that at the time of the Revolution there were not living in all the colonies 400 physicians who had received medical degrees; and yet, as is stated elsewhere, there were presumed to be over 3,500 practitioners. The American colleges had up to 1776 in the aggregate issued but fifty-one degrees, including that of bachelor of medicine. At the close of the century, those who had received degrees from American institutions did not number 250, but probably five times this number had attended one course of lectures at the different colleges, and who were then in practice. The colonists at first, it would seem, rather preferred to patronize the medical man who was also minister, farmer, merchant, or mechanic in addition to being a physician. Nor is it strange that a population in a new country, compelled to be industrious, frugal, and primitive in their habits, should welcome those who most nearly adopted their own mode of life. It will be remembered that there were neither medical clubs, institutions, quizzes, nor clinics to aid the medical student; and the libraries of medical men, as a general fact, contained but few works, and those were text-books of the most general character. There was, perhaps, not a medical library in the country prior to the Revolution that would have numbered 1,000 volumes and the vast majority of physicians did not have 50. From these facts the advantages, or rather want of advantages, of the early medical student may be inferred. The great majority of practitioners of medicine throughout the colonies down to the Revolution were never enabled to attend lectures, visit hospital-clinics, or, as it was termed, walk the hospital, for such institutions did not exist in this country. Students having concluded the term for which they engaged to read with a physician, they commenced their career as practitioners. The practice, however, was quite common for the student to study in the office of some physician enjoying a reputation for surgery or for the treatment of fevers, or specially noted for some branch of his profession, for a year or two, and then to go to the office of another who enjoyed a similar reputation for excellence in another branch; but the usage was general that the young physicians left the offices of their preceptors to commence practice. In but a few States were licenses or certificates required, and these were easily obtained. The doctor's office, too, at that period, had not the luxurious appointments of the present day. It was generally a one-story single room, joining or adjacent to the doctor's house; the exception was for it to have two rooms; these were kept in order by the students themselves. It was rarely plastered; was shelved around the walls to hold bottles and medicine and the few medical books the doctor's library contained. It was never carpeted and was too often cheerless in the extreme. It was neither inviting to the student nor to the patient, nor to their friends who had to visit it. The paraphernalia of saddle-bags, overcoats, buffalo-robes, and the usual outfit of the country doctor were almost everywhere obtrusively apparent about the room.

As the cabin preceded the comfortable farm-dwelling and the school-house and academy preceded the college, just so the primitive medical men preceded the more cultured and accomplished physicians of a later period. It will always follow that the higher and more general the standard of education in a country, the higher will be the standard of professional acquirements demanded by the public.

We have stated elsewhere that up to the beginning of the revolutionary war but two medical colleges had been organized in the United States.

The war of the Revolution gave great impetus and energy to the whole population of the colonies. The experience gained by the medical men who served in the Army elevated their views, gave them confidence in the exercise of their professional duties, endeared them to the public, and made them almost oracles in the communities in which they resided. This spirit of gratitude also created friends for the profession in the various legislatures, led to the enactment of laws which were more

[1] For political reasons the charter of the College of Philadelphia was abrogated in 1779, and the University of Pennsylvania chartered and a faculty organized. In 1789 the powers and privileges were restored to the College of Philadelphia, but leaving the university with its endowments from confiscated estates and all the powers at first granted. The two schools continued their separate course until the close of the year 1791. Whole number of graduates, including the bachelor and doctor's degree, from College of Philadelphia, from 1765 to its union with the university, 38. Whole number of graduates from the organization of University of Pennsylvania to the close of the century, 131.* The first medical college organized in New York was under the patronage of King's College in 1768; the chairs all became vacant in 1776. Up to this period there had been 14 graduates receiving the bachelor's or doctor's degree.† In 1787 the name of the college was changed to that of Columbia College and measures taken to organize a new faculty, which was not completed until 1792. From 1792-'93 to 1800 there were

* History of the Medical Department of the University of Pennsylvania, p. 218.
† Medical Register of the City of New York, 1862, p. 167.

just and protecting in their character and popularized the more recent and thorough modes for the scientific study of medicine. Hitherto dissections of the human body were very offensive to the public sentiment, but the war greatly lessened this prejudice, and the last vestige of this opposition manifested itself in 1788 in New York, and from that time forward medical schools have not been interfered with in using in a proper way fitting subjects in the dissecting-room. From this period, also, may be dated the greatest liberality on the part of the law-makers for the encouragement of medical colleges, medical societies, and curative institutions. This of itself inspired the ambition of youths in every community to enter a profession that was so honored, and there to win distinction. During the period from the close of the Revolution to the beginning of the present century, there was a marked increase of medical students in the country, and no less than five additional colleges, or rather medical faculties, organized; but in 1800 we find only four of them in actual existence, welcoming within them the medical students of America. From the beginning of the present century, the number of our medical students who went to Europe to complete their education became fewer. The colleges, too, were increasing the number of distinct chairs or professorships and the facilities for the student were being increased. The number of medical works that were being published in the country was noticeably on the increase, many of them being printed at interior towns of the different States, where since 1800 scarcely any book had been published. It is true that these publications were chiefly, and often with comments, editions of French and English works. Few original ones, up to the close of the last century, were made by American authors; and up to the close of the century but one original medical journal was published in the country.

INTERRUPTION FROM WAR.

The promising career of these institutions was early interrupted by the stirring events which ushered in the Revolution.

---

in this school 225 matriculants and 15 M. D. graduates.* In 1787 Nicholas Romayne established a respectable private medical school and continued it as such until 1791 without issuing degrees, when he associated with him a few others. They first applied for recognition and powers to grant degrees from the University of New York. This not being granted, they accepted powers from Queen's (now Rutgers) College of New Jersey, in 1793.† I am n ot able to state what number graduated from this school; but, as the organization was not long continued, there were but very few. The medical faculty of Harvard University, up to the close of the century, granted but 9 medical diplomas.‡ Dartmouth Medical College, which organized its medical faculty in 1796, up to the close of the century had granted but 5 medical degrees.§ The whole number of medical degrees granted by all seven of these medical faculties, up to the close of the eighteenth century, amounted to only about 212.

* Inaugural Discourse, Rutgers College, by Hosack, p. 85.
† Manley's Address as President of the New York Medical Society, 1827.
‡ College Catalogue.
§ College Catalogue.

Political excitement and the preparations for war claimed the attention of the citizens. *Inter arma silent doctores.* Some of the professors continued to impart instruction for a time and none were indifferent to the struggle, while most of those who were natives of this country received important commissions either from the colonial or Federal Government.

Since the establishment of American independence, when we had less than 4,000,000 population and but two medical colleges, these institutions have so multiplied in the land, that now, with a population of perhaps 40,000,000, there is scarcely a State that has not one or more flourishing medical schools. In the aggregate there are now over one hundred medical teaching bodies in the United States. The classes attending these various colleges number about 7,000, with an annual list of graduates of over 2,000.

The author wishes to acknowledge the assistance of Dr. R. M. Wyckoff in the preparation of this article.

ALPHABETICAL INDEX TO NAMES OF PHYSICIANS MENTIONED IN THE TEXT.

A.

Name	Page.
Adams, David	69
Adams, Henry	35
Adams, Samuel	35, 44
Adams, William	83
Ahl, John Peter	89
Alcock, John	18
Alcock, Samuel	18
Alcocke, N.	15
Alexander, Nathaniel	64
Allen, Daniel	19
Allison, Richard	83
Alsop, J	15
Ames, Nathaniel	25
Ames, Seth	29
Applewhaite, John	93
Appleton, Nathaniel Walker	24
Archer, John	88
Arents, Jacob	73
Arnold, Jonathan	71
Aspinwall, William	23
Attwood, Dr.	45, 58
Atwater, David	65
Austin, Caleb	46
Avery, Jonathan	19
Avery, William	18
Axon, Samuel J.	62
Aylef, J	15
Ayrault, Pierre	70

B.

Name	Page.
Bacon, General	9
Bagnall, Anthony	8
Bailey, Dr.	100
Baird, Absalom	80, 83
Baker, James	28
Baker, Moses	32
Baldwin, Cornelius	10
Ballantine, Eban	35
Barber, Luke	87
Bard, John	44, 73, 104
Bard, Samuel	44, 57, 101
Barnaby, Ruth	18
Barnet, Oliver	76
Barnet, William	76, 77
Baron, Alexander	63

Name	Page.
Bartlett, Daniel	35
Bartlett, John	72
Bartlett, Josiah	33, 49, 100, 101
Bartlett, Moses	65, 68
Bartlett, Moses, jr	68
Barret, Dr.	23
Barrett, Daniel	76
Bartram, John	79
Bass, John	72
Baxter, Joseph	26
Bayley, Richard	45
Baylies, William	28
Baynham, John	11
Baynham, William	11
Beal, Dr.	18
Beatty, Reading	83
Bedford, Nathaniel	81
Beekman, Gerardus	39, 49
Belcher, Dr.	25
Belcher, E	68
Beltsnyder, William	38
Bellingham, Samuel	12
Berry, Thomas	31
Binney, Barnabas	31
Bird, John	67
Bloomfield, Moses	77
Blyth, Joseph	64
Bodo, Otto	77
Bogart, Nicholas N	72
Bohun, Lawrence	8
Bond, Thomas	83, 84, 85, 98
Booerhaave, Dr.	96
Bowen, Elijah	73
Bowen, Elijah, jr	74
Bowen, Ephraim	70, 72
Bowen, Joseph	72
Bowen, Pardon	72
Bowen, Richard	71
Boyd, John	89
Boylston, Thomas	16
Boylston, Zabdiel	22
Brackett, Joshua	100
Bradford, William	71
Bredewardyn, William	15
Brehm, James	63
Bret, John	70
Brett, Robert	42

INDEX.

Name	Page
Brewer, James	43
Brickett, James	93
Bringham, Origen	35
Brinley, Frank	43
Brooks, Dr.	35
Brown, Benjamin	72
Brown, Ezekiel	35
Brown, Gustavus	88
Brown, Gustavus	88
Brown, Jabez	70
Brown, Jabez, jr	70
Brown, James	83
Brown, Joseph	70
Brownfield, Robert	62
Brownson, Nathan	62
Brunson, Isaac	69
Buchanan, George	87
Buckman, Nathan	30
Budd, Bernard	76
Budd, John C.	76
Bulkley, John	26, 67
Bull, Ezekiel	12
Bull, William	61
Bulfinch, Thomas	23, 24
Bulfinch, Thomas, jr	23
Bullivant, Benjamin	19
Burnet, Ichabod	77
Burnet, William	77
Butler, William	63
Butts, William	15

C.

Cabell, William	9
Cadwallader, Thomas	46, 79, 84
Caldwell, Andrew	83
Calvert, Jonathan	11, 90
Campbell, George, of New Jersey	75
Campbell, George, of New York	46
Campbell, Dr.	66
Campfield, Jabez	77
Carne, John	62
Carrington, Elias	66
Carroll, Charles	88
Carter, Ezra	100
Carter, James	11
Carter, William	11
Castine, Abel	66
Chace, John	72
Chalmers, Lionel	61, 63
Chambre, John	15, 16
Chancy, Isaac	13
Chauncy, Charles	13
*Cheever, Abijah	35
*Cherts, Michiel de Marco	39
Child, Robert	18

Name	Page
Child, Timothy	34
Chrystie, Thomas	10, 11
Church, Benjamin	23, 33
Clark, Dr., of Massachusetts	104
Clark, John, of Rhode Island	70
Clarke, John, of Massachusetts	14
Clarke, John, jr., of Massachusetts	14
Claude, Dennis	87
Clayton, John	11
Clayton, Joshua	92
Clements, Mace	10
Clossy, Samuel	45, 97, 101
Cochran, John	46, 47, 77
Coggeswell, William	35, 100
Cogswell, Mason Fitch	66
Colden, Cadwallader	42, 49
Coleman, Asaph	68
Coleman, Noah	69
Commer, Jacob D.	39
Condict, John	75, 76
Cook, Samuel	46
Cooke, Elisha	22
Cooke, Elisha, jr	22
Cooke, Stephen	11
Corbett, John	24, 28
Corbett, John, jr	24
Cornelius, Elias	46
Coulter, Dr.	89
Courts, Richard Henry	89
Cox, Daniel	73
Craddock, Dr.	89
Cragie, Andrew	46
Craik, James	10
Crane, John	35
Cranston, John	70
Craven, Gersham	74
Creed, Dr.	76
Crosby, Ebenezer	43
Crossman, George	27
Crouch, Dr.	27
Cullen, Dr.	96
Currie, James	11
Curtis, Alexander C.	39
Curtis, Benjamin	23
Curtis, Samuel, of New Hampshire	101
Curtis, Samuel, of North Carolina	64
Cushing, Lemuel	35
Cutler, John	23
Cutter, Ammi	25
Cutting, John B.	92

D.

Name	Page
Dalhounde, Lawrence	23, 24
Danforth, Elijah	24, 25
Danforth, Samuel	31, 33

INDEX.

	Page.		Page.
Darby, Henry White	75	Flint, Edward	26
Darby, John, of Connecticut	69	Forman, Aaron	76
Darby, John, of New Jersey	75	Foster, Isaac	93
Davidson, James	83	Fothergill, Dr.	85
Davis, Jonathan	28	Francis, John W	42
Davis, Joseph	10	Francis, John	16
Dean, Ezra	26	Franklin, Benjamin	9, 44
Deancy, Dr.	74	Frunk, John	35
Deeping, William	38	Fuller, Jabez	34
De Hinse, Dr.	40	Fuller, Matthew	13
Denwood, Levin	90	Fuller, Samuel	12
Dexter, Aaron	31	Fries, Jaques	15
Dexter, William	26	**G.**	
Dickinson, John	66, 68	Gager, William	12
Dickinson, Jonathan	73	Gale, Benjamin	23, 67, 68
Doggett, Ebenezer	26	Galt, John Minson	11
Douglass, William	22	Gardiner, Jos	23, 24
Drake, Daniel	104	Gardiner, Sylvester	23, 71
Draper, George	46	Gardiner, William	79
Druce, John	27	Gardner, Alexander	61
Dubois, Isaac	42	Gardner, Samuel	30
Duffield, John	35	Gelston, Samuel	23
Du Parck, Jan	39	Gerrard, Dr.	86
Dupuy, John	42	Gilder, Reuben	92
E.		Glentworth, George	80
Edmonston, Samuel	90	Glover, John	13
Egbert, Jacob V	93	Glover, Samuel Kingsley	32
Elbert, John L	90	Goldineau, Giles	40
Eliot, Jared	65, 66, 67	Goddard, T	15
Elliott, John	46	Godfrey, Philip	23
Elmer, Ebenezer	75	Goforth, Dr.	104
Elmer, Jonathan	74, 76	Goodson, John	78
Elmer, Moses	77	Goodwin, Francis Le Baron	35
Ely, John	67	Goss, Eben Harden	34
Erving, Shirley	33	Gott, Benjamin	31
Eustis, William	32	Gould, David	11
Evans, Cadwallader	79, 84	Gould, Witham	69
Evertsen, Arent	40	Graeme, Thomas	79
Ewing, Thomas	74	Graham, Andrew	44
		Graham, Isaac Gilbert	35, 44
F.		Graham, Stephen	46
Fayssoux, Peter	62	Graham, William	11
Fereis, B	15	Graves, Thomas	23
Fergus, James	64	Gray, Dr	89
Finley, James B. C	35	Green, Ezra	93, 101
Finley, Samuel	35	Green, Dr	9
Firmin, Giles	12, 64	Green, James W	64
Fisher, Adam	90	Griffin, Corbin	12, 93
Fisher, Daniel	34	Griffin, Cyrus	12
Fisk, John	12	Griffith, David	12
Fisk, Joseph	35	Griffith, John	77
Fisk, Phineas	65, 68	Griffith, Owen	79
Fiske, Henry	91	Gulstone, Dr.	8
Flagg, Henry C	62	Gunn, Frederick	62

INDEX.

H.

	Page.
Hale, Elizur	68
Hale, Elizur, jr	68
Hale, Mordecai	46
Haliburton, Dr	70
Hall, Jeremiah	30
Hall, Lyman	49, 63
Hall, Percival	35
Hallewell, Nicholas	16
Halsted, Robert	74
Halsted, Caleb	75
Hamilton, Dr	84
Hanie, Ezekiel	90
Hanna, John	75
Harding, Jos	12
Harman, E	15
Harris, Robert	83
Harris, Tucker	63
Harris, Jacob	77
Harrison, Elisha	90
Hart, John	93
Hart, Oliver	62
Haslet, Dr	89
Hastings, Walter	35, 93
Hastings, Dr., of Connecticut	69
Hays, William	38
Hayward, Lemuel	30
Hewes, Jos	71
Hewins, Elijah	30
Hewins, Lemuel	30
Hitchcock, Gad	29
Hoar, Leonard	12
Hobart, Peter	34
Hobbs, William	15
Hodgson, Dr	78
Holbrook, Amos	33
Holden, Phineas	30
Holden, William	25, 30
Holling, Solomon	64
Holmes, David	69
Holten, Samuel	28
Holyoke, Edw. Augustus	31
Homans, John	24
Horner, Gustavus Brown	90
Hosmer, Timothy	69
Houston, James	62, 93
Howell, Lewis	75
Hubbard, Laurett	69
Hughes, Joseph, of New York	39
Hughes, Joseph, of Rhode Island	27
Hughes, William	22
Hulse, Dr	89
Hunt, Ebenezer	29
Hunter, William	70
Hurlburt, James	65
Husbands, Edward	87
Hutchinson, Ebenezer	46
Hutchinson, James	80
Hutchinson, Mrs	18

I.

	Page.
Irvine, William	80

J.

Jacobs, Jos	27
Jackson, Clement	25, 100
Jackson, David	80
Jackson, Hall	100
Jamison, Dr	82
Jansen, Isaac	38
Jarvis, Charles	24
Jennifer, Daniel	91
Jepson, William	67
Jerauld, James	25
Jerauld, James, jr	25, 29
Johnson, James	76
Johnson, Lancelot	64
Johnson, Robert	83
Johnson, Samuel	76
Johnson, Uzal	75
Jones, David	93
Jones, Edward	78
Jones, Evan	46, 78, 79
Jones, James	92
Jones, John	45, 83, 101
Jones, Margaret	17
Jones, Walter	12

K.

Kast, Philip Godfrist	31
Kast, Thomas	31
Kearsley, John	44, 79, 104
Keene, Samuel Y	90
Kellogg, Giles Crouch	27
Kennedy, Patrick	90
Kent, Richard	15
Kerfbyle, Johannes	40, 57
Kierstede, Hans	38, 39
Kilty, William	90
Kirkpatrick, Dr	61
Kittredge, Tho	35
Kittridge, Thomas	29
Knight, John	93
Kollock, Cornelius	33
Kuhn, Adam Simon	79, 82
Kuhn, Adam	82, 98

L.

Ladley, Andrew	83
Lajournade, Alex	90
La Montague, Johannes	38, 40

INDEX.

Name	Page
Land, Charles	10
Latimer, Henry	92
Laughlin, William	35
Leavenworth, Thomas	65
Ledyard, Isaac	46
Lee, Daniel	71
Lee, Samuel	69
Le Baron, Francis	19
Le Baron, Joseph	34
Le Baron, Lazarus	34
Le Baron, Lazarus, jr	34
Leiper, Andrew	10
Lindere, Thomas	16
Lining, John	61
Little, Thomas	24
Lloyd, James	23, 27, 29, 58, 104
Lockhart, Dr	40
Lockman, Charles	62
Lockman, John	63, 84
Logan, George	81
L'Orange, Jacob	39
Lord, Dr	23
Loughton, William	35
Love, David	64
Lowthrain, Thomas	31
Lumbrozo, Jacob	86
Lynn, John	35
Lyon, William	87, 89

M.

McCalla, Thomas	83
McCarter, Charles	84
McClure, William	64
McClurg, Walter	10
McClurg, James	11
McCoffrey, Samuel A	83
McCosky, Alex	83
McDonald, Archibald	43
McDowell, John	83
McFarlin, Dr	76
McHenry, James	89
McKean, Robert	77
McKinly, John	91
McKnight, Charles	43
McLain, William	64
McLelland, Dr	82
Macry, Robert	11
Magaw, William	83
Malcolm, Henry	84
Mallenacy, Jacob	38
Mann, James	34, 90
Manlove, Christopher	77
Mans, Matthew	83
Marion, Jos	23

Name	Page
Marsh, Dr	34
Martin, Ennals	91
Martin, Hugh	83
Martin, James	62
Mather, Timothy	69
Mattel, Louis	63
Matthews, Andrew	13
Maubray, John	58, 61
Mawney, John	70
Maynadier, Henry	91
Megapolensis, Samuel	38, 39
Menema, Daniel	46
Mercer, Hugh	10
Metcalf, John	27
Michlau, Paul	77
Middleton, Baziel	10, 73, 101
Middleton, Peter	44, 45
Millengen, Dr	63
Miller, Edward	91
Miller, John	92
Miller, Seth	45
Mitchell, Alex	88, 91
Mitchell, John	9, 10
Moffatt, Thomas	70
Molenaer, Dr	40
Monforde, J.	15
Monroe, George	10, 92
Monroe, Thomas	72
Moore, Henry	46
Moore, Nicholas	80
Moore, Samuel Preston	80
Moores, Abijah	65
Morgan, Abel	84
Morgan, Benjamin	35
Morgan, John	58, 74, 78, 81, 96, 99
Morrison, Norman	65
Morrow, David	90
Morrow, Samuel	90
Morse, Isaac	76
Mosely, Isaac	67
Moultrie, John	58, 61
Moway, Peter	81
Munson, Eneas	68
Munroe, Stephen	81
Murray, James	89

N.

Nelson, John	88
Neufville, William	62
Nichols, Christopher	72
Nicholson, Robert	84
Nicoll, John	42
Noyes, John	67, 69
Noyes, Oliver	19

INDEX.

O.

	Page.
Oaks, Thomas	22
Ogden, Jacob	44, 45
Oliphant, David	62, 63
Oliver, Thomas	13
Ordway, Dr	100
Orne, Jos	30
Osborne, John	44, 67
Osborne, John, jr	67
Osborne, Samuel	44
Otis, Isaac	25
Owens, Griffith	78
Owens, Samuel	87

P.

	Page.
Packer, Dr	100
Parish, John	72
Parker, William	100
Patridge, Oliver	31
Patterson, Robert	77
Pau, John	38
Pecker, James	29
Pecker, James, jr	29
Peet, Abraham	65
Peirson, Abraham	73
Peirson, Mathias	77
Pen, J	15
Peres, Peter J	83
Perkins, John	23
Perkins, Jos	66
Perkins, Nathaniel	23
Perkins, William Lee	23
Perry, Dr	67
Phelps, Elisha	68
Phillips, Nathaniel	19
Pierce	100
Pigot, Edward	77
Pindell, Richard	90
Pinquerou, N. T	73
Piltersen, Evart	40
Platt, Samuel	83
Pope, John	24
Porter, Daniel	66
Pot, John	8, 49
Potter, James	67
Potter, Jared	69
Potts, Jonathan	99
Pratt, John	13
Pratt, Shuball	11
Prentice Dr	81
Prescott, Jos	62
Prescott, Oliver	26
Prescott, Oliver, jr	26
Prince, Jonathan	28
Prior, Abner	46

	Page.
Pue Dr	89
Putnam, Amos	29
Pynchon, Charles	23, 29

R.

	Page.
Ramsey, David	61
Ramsey, Jesse H	62
Ramsey, John	84
Rand, Isaac	23, 29, 33
Rand, Isaac, jr	29
Rawson, Eliot	65
Read, William	62, 63
Redman, Thomas	71
Redman, John	80, 81, 82, 83, 104
Reed, Thomas	46, 47
Reineck, Christian	84
Reinick, Christopher	84
Rhodes, Jos	72
Richards, Benjamin	25
Richards, Jos	24
Richardson, Abijah	31
Richmond, Ebenezer	72
Ridgely, Charles	91
Roberts, Aaron	68, 69
Roberts, John	11, 23, 93
Rockhill, John	73
Rodman, Thomas	72
Rogers, Daniel	25
Rogers, John	13, 25, 84
Rogers, John R. B	84
Rogers, Nathaniel	100
Rogne, John	83
Romayne, Nicholas	45, 108
Rose, John	67, 69
Rose, Josiah	67
Rose, Robert	10, 63
Rumney, William	12
Rush, Benjamin	9, 49, 82, 91, 99, 104
Rush, Jos	63
Russell, Walter	8

S.

	Page.
Sackett, Samuel	84
Sage, Ebenezer	44
Salstonstall, Henry	12
Samon, X	15
Saple, John A	83
Sargent, Nathaniel	100
Savage, Jos	10
Savil, Elisha	29
Sawyer, Micajah	27
Scammel, John	28
Scammel, Samuel Leslie	27
Scammel, Samuel Leslie, jr	28
Scarborough, Sir Charles	16

INDEX.

	Page.
Schult, Gerrett	38
Schuyler, Nicholas	46, 47
Seabury, Samuel	13
Senter, Isaac	7
Shaaf, John T.	89
Sharpe, James B.	93
Shepard, David	47
Shippen, Wm.	78, 81, 82, 84, 96, 97, 99, 102
Shippen, William, jr.	58, 82
Shults, John Gerard	73
Shute, Daniel	35
Shute, Samuel Moore	76
Simpson, John	67, 69
Skeele, Amos	69
Skinner, Alex	10
Skinner, Elisha	93
Skinner, Thomas	69
Smith, Alexander	90
Smith, Clement	90
Smith, Elihu Hubbard	66, 91
Smith, Isaac	69
Smith, James	88
Smith, John	89, 90, 101
Smith, Nathan	10
Smith, William	83
Smith, William P.	46
Somerville, William	89
Spaulding, Lyman	56
Spencer, John	10
Sprague, John	24
Springer, Sylvester	62
Staats, Abraham	38
Staats, Samuel	39
Starr, Comfort	12
Starrs, Thomas	13
Steadman, Edward	26
Stenhouse Dr.	89
Stevens, William S.	62
Stevenson, George	83, 92
Stevenson, Henry	87, 88
Stevenson, John	87
Stewart, Alex	83
Stockett, Thomas Noble	88
Stockbridge, Benjamin	24, 27
Stockbridge, Charles	27
Stockton, Benjamin	46, 77
Stone, Samuel	22
Storrs, Justus	69
Stringer, Samuel	47
Strippe, Roger	15
Stuber, Henry	78
Snagent, Nathaniel	100
Sumner, Enos	30
Sutton, Edward	65

	Page.
Swain, Thomas	34
Sweet, Caleb	46
Swett, John Barnard	32
Sykes, James	92
Symson, N	15

T.

Tabbs, Barton	89
Taylor, Charles	12
Taylor, Christopher	83
Taylor, Henry	22, 39
Tennant, John V. B	101
Tenny, Samuel	72
Tetard, Benjamin	62, 93
Texier, Felix	93
Thacher, James	33
Thacher, Peter	22
Thacher, Thomas	19
Thayer, Jonathan	25
Thomas, John	35, 43, 47
Thomas, Philip	89
Thomas, William	35
Thompson, Benjamin	18
Thompson, Jos	83
Thompson, Thad	35
Thornbill, Thomas	42
Thornton, Matthew	49
Throop, Amos	72
Tilden, John	90
Tillotson, Thomas	90
Tilton, James	92, 99
Touton, John	19
Townsend, David	35, 93
Treadwell, Benjamin	45
Treat, Malachi	46
Tresvant, John	10
Tucker, Thomas T	62
Tufts, Cotton	26
Tufts, Simon	26
Tunison, Garrett	77
Turner, Daniel	66
Turner, Henry	25
Turner, Henry, jr	25
Turner, Peter	72
Turner, William	73
Tylby, W	15

U.

Usher, Robert	69

V.

Vacher, John F	46
Van Beuren, Beekman	42
Van Beuren, John	42
Van de Bogaerdet, Herman M	38

INDEX.

Name	Page.
Vanden Berg, Peter Jansen	39
Van der Lynn, Peter	46
Van Dyck, Cornelius	39
Van Eflinchoone, Lucal	42
Vanevanger, Dr.	39
Van Imbroeck, Gysbert	39
Van Rosenburgh, William	41
Van Wagenner, Garrett	83
Varvanger, Jacob Henrickson	38
Vaughn, Claiborne	10, 63
Von Belcamp, Jacob	39
Veisselius, George Andrew	74
Vicary, Thomas	15
Vickers, Samuel	62
Victoria, Fernandes de	16
Vigneron, Charles Antonius	71
Vigneron, Norbert Felician	71
Vreucht, Peter	23

W.

Name	Page.
Waldo, Albigeren	69
Wales, Ephraim	29
Walker, George	87
Walker, James	87
Wallace, James	10
Wallace, John	62
Ward, Samuel	74
Ward, Seth	74
Ware, Benjamin	19
Warfield, Charles Alex	88
Warfield, Walter	90
Warren, John	65
Warren, Joseph	30, 32, 65
Warren, Petetiah	100
Waters, Wilson	90
Watrous, John R	67, 69
Watrous, Josiah	46
Weisenthall, Dr	89
Welch, Thomas	34
Welles, Benjamin	47
Wentworth, Miles	23
Wessels, Herman	39
West, Benjamin	70
Wharry, Robert	83
Wheaton, Levi	72
Wheeler, William	46

Name	Page.
Whimple, Walter Vrooman	47
Whipple, Jos	24
Whipple, Daniel Peck	72
White, Ebenezer	43
White, Nathaniel	19, 30
Whitewell, Samuel	35
Whiting, William	26
Whitworth, M	23
Wilkins, John	80, 83
Willard, Moses	47
Williams, John D	76
Williams, Nathaniel	22
Williams, Obadiah	93
Williams, Robert	64
Williams, Samuel	29
Williamson, Hugh	63
Wilson, John	14, 26
Wislon, John, jr	26
Wilson, Matthew	91
Wilson, Robert	63
Wilson, Samuel	63
Wingate, John	93
Winslow, Edward,	18
Winthrop, John	35
Winthrop, John, jr	35
Wistar, Caspar	83
Witt, Christopher	79
Wolcott, Oliver	49, 66
Wood, Gerard	90
Wood, Thomas	73
Woodruff, Aaron	83
Woodruff, Henlock	46
Woodruff, Samuel	46
Wooten, Thomas	8
Worthington, Charles	90
Wright, Aaron	29
Wright, John G	93
Wynn, Thomas	78

Y.

Name	Page.
Yates, George	10
Yearly, Robert	16
Young, Joseph	46
Younglove, Moses	47

Z.

Name	Page.
Zachary, Lloyds	79